Second edition

Coach Yourself to
Wellness

Living The Intentional Life

Fiona Cosgrove

Cosgrove, Fiona.
Coach yourself to wellness : living the intentional life / author, Fiona Cosgrove.

1st ed.
2nd ed.
ISBN-13: 978-0-646-80551-1

Bibliography.
Health.
Well-being.

Published by Wellness Coaching Australia
www.wellnesscoachingaustralia.com.au

Coach Yourself to
Wellness

Living The Intentional Life

Fiona Cosgrove

*Create lasting change in your fitness, weight
control, nutrition and stress management*

Second edition

How to use this book

Scan through the book.

Go back and read it carefully. Some sections will "speak" to you more than others. Read them twice.

Start to think about what you would like to change and what you could do to take the first steps.

You may be already in the change process for some parts of your wellness. The book may help move you forward in other areas.

When you are ready to begin, consider using the Coach Yourself to Wellness Workbook that is available with the text. It will give you a concrete guide for you (or your clients) to use and help keep you on track.

Never forget to enlist all the help you need. There are many different ways of getting it and you will be surprised at how readily available it is! And you will be surprised how many other people are facing the same challenges as you.

If you would like a coach and/or a trainer, contact: info@ wellnesscoachingaustralia.com.au

Or go to www.wellnesscoachingaustralia.com.au

Believe in yourself!

Dedication

To the many people who have worked with me over the last decade or so to help me create my business. The birth of the new industry of health and wellness coaching both in Australia and internationally takes time, effort and belief in what we do. It could never be done alone. Thank you to my colleagues and my family for your love and support.

About the Author

Fiona Cosgrove is one of
Australia's most esteemed
wellness coaches. She has been
involved in the health and
fitness industry for over 30 years,
creating health clubs in Asia
and Australia that offer so much
more than purely equipment and
classes. With two Masters degrees in sports science and counselling,
Fiona understands the connection between exercise prescription,
health knowledge and action-orientated coaching. Fiona believes
passionately in people's ability to become their 'best self' and the
importance of wellness coaching as a new profession. With this in
mind, Fiona is leading the field in Australia, gaining recognition for
the need and value of health and wellness coaches to work towards
improving the mental and physical wellbeing of our communities.
She is also undertaking doctorate studies examining the effect of
coach training on the students who wish to work in this field. Her
other activities include speaking to various industries on topics
including motivation, confidence, improving wellness and energy
management.

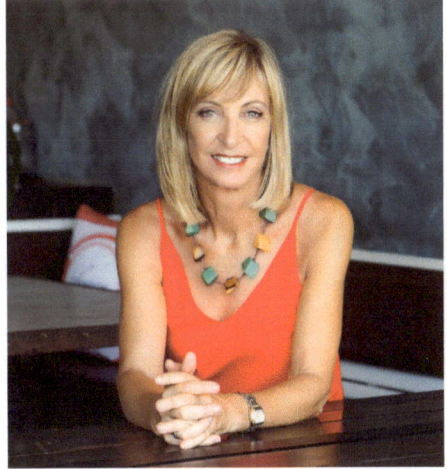

www.wellnesscoachingaustralia.com.au

Contents

Section 3 Changing behaviour   49

Section 4 The journey   75

Foreword

When it comes to finding our way on the path to wellness, it's not a surprise that many of us stumble or get stuck. For the first time in the era of modern medicine, we are being challenged to plot our own course.

While the idea of steering our own wellness ships fits with our urges for self-determination, on the whole we lack the tools, skills and experience to get out of the harbour. In the face of a map-less journey, how do we find the guide rails to support us for the long haul?

I first met Fiona Cosgrove when she enrolled in Wellcoaches training and her excitement was infectious. Her work with clients in Sydney was synergistic with the Wellcoaches coaching psychology model. She was keen to spread the word about the power of wellness coaching. We share an unwavering commitment to guiding people to develop the life skills they need to take charge of their own wellness. Fiona also inspires our commitment for Wellcoaches to reach every corner of the globe so that wherever there are people who want to gain mastery of their health and well-being, there will be qualified coaches to support them.

If you want to make lasting and meaningful changes in your life, Coach Yourself to Wellness is an essential guide. This book will show you how to create a wellness plan and bring it to life through commitment, action and self-belief.

Fiona Cosgrove has passion and talent for showing fellow travellers how to find their own wellness compasses. This book is a testament to both.

Margaret Moore
Founder and CEO, Wellcoaches Corporation
Wellesley, MA, USA

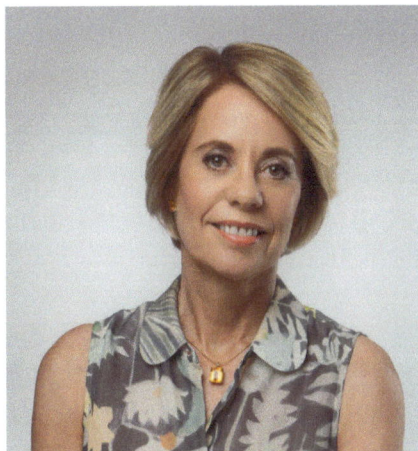

Introduction

This book is about vibrancy and energy and growth. It is not about finding inner calm, although you may well achieve that. After 25 years of working in the fitness industry, watching people succeed (sometimes) and relapse or fail (many more times) I knew there had to be something we could offer other than expert advice.

People know what to do in order to lose weight, get fit and destress; they just don't know how to do it. I became very interested in the underlying reasons that were stopping clients from making permanent change in their health and wellbeing. Coaching people towards their own goals seemed to have more effect than telling people what to do. Coaching psychology theory and in particular, positive psychology, had a great influence on my way of thinking and I started to see things shift for clients. I began to see that once clients took responsibility for their change process, they had greater commitment and success.

I then discovered Wellcoaches who had a clearly defined and researched model that incorporated much of what I had been doing and the path became much clearer. I was able to slowly build my own training business for the Australian market and take it further. The years have gone by, and having trained several thousand people, Wellness Coaching Australia is an established business with a strong reputation for being a leader in the field.

We welcome change and growth and look forward to building a community of coaches and training organisations who can in turn help others create their best lives.

I have enormous respect and admiration for people who want to make change and are willing to take the first step. Because that is how it is done: one small step after another, slowly moving forward. Transformation can happen but it rarely happens overnight. It takes time, effort and commitment to change ingrained habits. But new habits can be developed and with the right tools, a different life can unfold. And with optimal wellness, that life can be anything you want it to be.

I thank everyone who has been involved in creating this wonderful industry and all the many people I have coached over the last 12 years who gave me the certainty to write this book. I know that each of us has what it takes to make our lives truly well and wonderful - often we just need a little help along he way. I hope that this book can provide support and encouragement on your journey of change.

Fiona Cosgrove,
Founder and CEO of Wellness Coaching Australia
Queensland, Australia

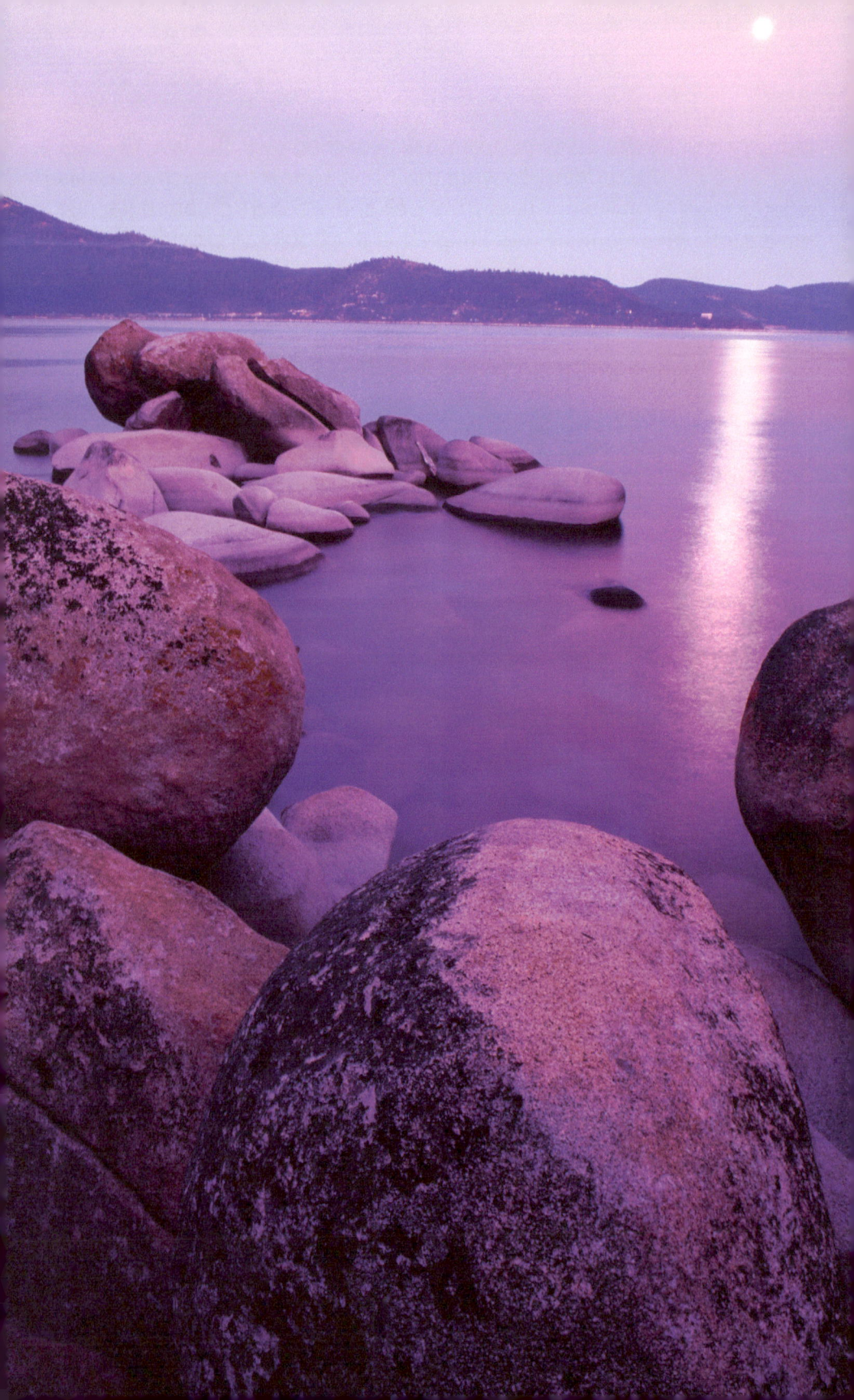

Section one

WELLNESS COACHING

What is wellness?

There are probably as many definitions of wellness as there are people using the term. The concept has different meanings for different people, mainly because the experience of being well is so subjective. Ranging from "the absence of disease" to "living life well – as opposed to badly", the word wellness conjures up so much.

For the purposes of this book, let's assume that wellness refers to the best we can be emotionally, physically, mentally and spiritually. This way we are striving and moving towards a positive, rather than avoiding or moving away from a negative.

"Wellness is the process of becoming aware of and making choices toward a more successful existence." The National Wellness Institute

How do we achieve wellness?

Put simply, we achieve wellness through a series of steps that allow us to take control in a program of action that will lead us to the desired state. Along the way we design and act on behaviours that match our goals.

An effective wellness program should encompass diet, exercise, stress management and health.

Smoking

Tobacco smoking is responsible for 7.9% of the burden on the health of Australians. In 2004, 2.9 million Australians smoked daily but this is declining. Smoking is a major risk factor for coronary heart disease.

Inactivity

50% of Australian adults are not undertaking sufficient physical activity, and inactivity is highest among 30-59 year olds.

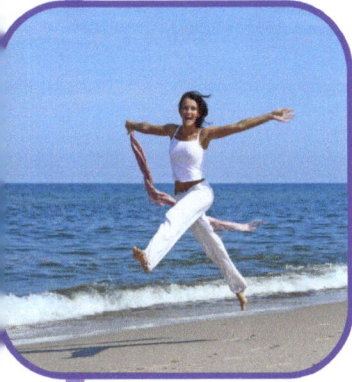

Why all the fuss about being well?

Several factors have led to the growth of this fledgling industry. Among them is growing awareness of:

- the large number of lifestyle-related illnesses and how they impact on our lives;

- the many different ways of living we can choose;

- the idea that life can be fulfilling and it is within our power to make it that way;

- the truth that happiness and wellness are not privileges reserved for the wealthy;

- the enormous number of choices and decisions we make every day that contribute to our feeling good or not so good.

In short, more people are becoming aware of wellness because they are waking up to the facts.

Being well means different things to different people. Wellness conjures up phrases such as:

- Bursting out of your skin
- On top of the world
- Peaceful
- Fulfilled
- Energetic and empowered
- Challenged and excited by life

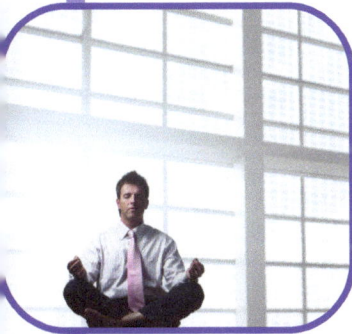

- In optimal health
- Fit and vital
- Able to deal with life's stresses
- Being in great shape
- Successful in life

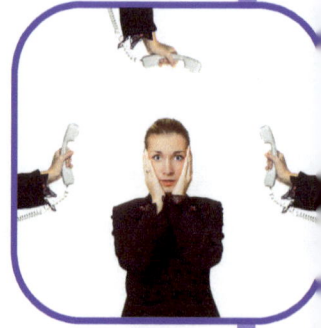

Obesity

Excess body fat increases the risk of developing a range of health problems including type 2 diabetes, cardiovascular disease, high blood pressure, certain cancers, sleep disorders, osteoarthritis, psychological disorders and social problems. Weight gain is essentially due to the energy intake from the diet being greater than the energy needed to fuel physical activity. Obesity levels have been on the rise and along with the United States, Canada and the United Kingdom, Australia is among the fattest countries in the world. The 2001 National Health Survey (NHS) showed 2.4 million Australian adults were estimated to be obese. A further 4.9 million Australian adults were estimated to be overweight but not obese. 20-25% of children and adolescents are overweight or obese.

High Blood Pressure

High blood pressure is a major risk factor for coronary heart disease, stroke, heart failure and kidney failure. The 1999 Australian Diabetes, Obesity and Lifestyle Study indicated that 30% of Australians (3.7 million) aged 25 years or older had high blood pressure. The best ways to treat high blood pressure are exercise and reducing stress.

So why aren't we *well* all the time?

Life is complex and demanding. Competing priorities often mean we don't make time to focus on what we want for ourselves - physically, mentally, emotionally and spiritually - or to create a plan to get there. This is where coaching can be incredibly supportive.

What is coaching?

The word coach has been used in many ways. Its associations with sport are probably strongest, but the traditional image of a forceful, demanding leader do not do the word justice. A more relevant way to describe coaching as it is practised across a range of disciplines would be:

A coach is a person who:

- Has expert knowledge but doesn't impose it on the person they are coaching
- Is a great role model but allows individual development of a person's talents and strengths
- Gives choices rather than orders
- Works with, rather than for
- Encourages and facilitates excellence and growth
- Measures their success in someone else's unique achievements.

Sound good?

It is.

We don't all have access to a good coach when we need one, but the good news is, it is possible to coach yourself. We just have to disable a few obstacles. One of our problems is that many of us have developed something in our personalities that works to destroy our confidence. Let's call it the inner anti-coach.

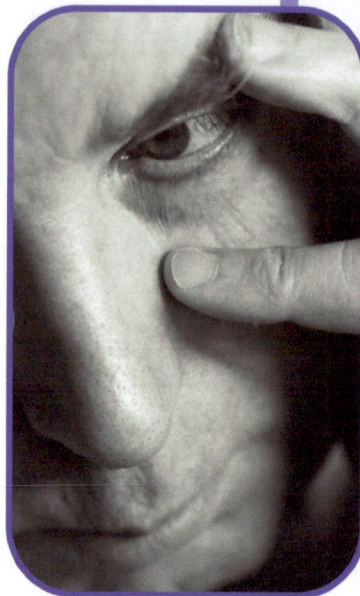

It seems to be that most human beings are hypersensitive to our own shortcomings. We know all too well when we have done something badly – when we've made a mistake, failed to achieve a goal or not met our own standards. Sometimes just looking in the mirror and not seeing perfection is enough. And the criticism starts. An inner voice berates us for our mistakes and flaws with labels that damn and demoralise.

Nutrition

Fruit and vegetable consumption is strongly linked to the prevention of chronic disease and to better health. Dietary guidelines recommend that adults consume 2-4 serves of fruit a day and 4-8 serves of vegetables per day. The 2004-05 National Health Survey showed that 85.7% of people aged 18 years or over did not usually consume the recommended quantity of vegetables and 46% did not consume two serves of fruit.

"How stupid can you be?" "Why must you always do things wrong?" "I knew you couldn't do it." "What is wrong with you?"

Sound familiar?

It's time to make a change and become your own Wellness coach. We will return to the inner anti-coach later.

Who uses coaching?

Strangely enough, it seems the people who have worked with a coach are not the people in greatest need of help. They usually are self-motivated and know they want to change. So if the idea of having a coach appeals to you, but there is something that is getting in the way right now, then this book is meant for you.

Excessive Alcohol Consumption

Excessive alcohol consumption is a major risk factor for morbidity and mortality. In Australia, in 1998-1999, the total tangible cost attributed to alcohol consumption was estimated at $5.5 billion (includes lost productivity, health care costs, road accident-related costs and crime related costs). (Collins and Lapsley, 2002.)

What is wellness coaching?

A wellness coach will work with their clients to identify areas for change that will lead to improved health, vitality and a greater sense of wellbeing. This may be different for each individual and the choice and responsibility for both choosing and achieving their wellness goals lies with the client. The coach will act as a facilitator and support and help the client discover their reasons for change, the factors that have been stopping them and how to overcome them. The relationship is one of trust and collaboration.

Become your own wellness coach

You are now about to become your own wellness coach. You must first approach the role in a professional way and teach yourself to ignore any negative internal messages that can get in the way of your success. You must be willing to regain control of your choices and set goals that are engineered to give the outcome you want. You will take charge of your health and wellness and become proficient at providing your own encouragement and support. Use this book as a tool; a guide to a process that will make positive change easily achievable.

Messages to tell yourself:

I can change

I am a good self-supporter

I have resilience

I choose to create a healthy life

I have values I am living up to

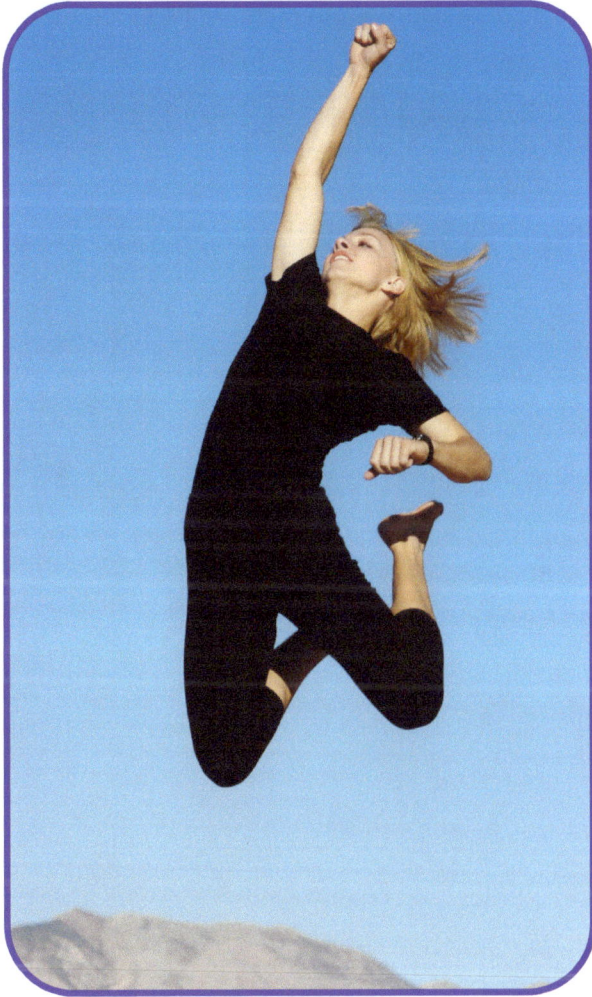

Beware! Common symptoms of wellness may include:

- Persistent presence of a support network
- Chronic positive expectations
- Episodic peak experiences
- Spiritual involvement
- Increased sensitivity
- Tendency to adapt to changing conditions
- Rapid recovery
- Increased appetite for physical activity
- Tendency to identify & communicate feelings
- Repeated episodes of gratitude and generosity
- Compulsion to contribute
- Persistent sense of humour

Cardiovascular Disease

Cardiovascular disease is the term used for heart, stroke and blood vessel diseases and is the leading cause of death in Australia. Cardiovascular disease kills one Australian every 10 minutes. According to the National Heart Foundation, many of these deaths are preventable. Arteries clog from excessive cholesterol and triglycerides which are a by-product of a high fat diet.

What is Health & Wellness Coaching?

Health and Wellness Coaches partner with clients seeking self-directed, lasting changes, aligned with their values, which promote health and wellness and, thereby, enhance well-being. In the course of their work health and wellness coaches display unconditional positive regard for their clients and a belief in their capacity for change, and honoring that each client is an expert on his or her life, while ensuring that all interactions are respectful and non-judgmental.

– National Board for Health and Wellness Coaching. (NBHWC)

Physical activity

- Reduces risk of cardiovascular problems
- Decreases chance of obesity and high blood pressure
- Increases HDL (good cholesterol)
- Decreases chance of type 2 diabetes
- Helps protect against some forms of cancer
- Strengthens musculoskeletal system
- Helps reduce chance of osteoporosis and risk of falls and fractures
- Improves mental wellbeing by reducing stress, anxiety and depression (in both the short and long term).

Summary

In this section we've learnt that:

- **Wellness is a subjective experience that involves moving towards optimal physical, mental, emotional and spiritual health.**

- **Wellness is achieved by creating a program of choices and strategies around diet, exercise, stress management, health maintenance and disease prevention.**

- **In Australia, the growing interest in being well is a response to the enormous evidence of our ill-health. Australians are waking up to the facts.**

- **The main reason we are not well all the time is our inability (or unwillingness) to prioritise wellness.**

- **Coaching is a supportive process that facilitates the achievement of goals through encouragement and accountability.**

- **Coaching can help counter the inner anti-coach – the voice that highlights all our shortcomings.**

- **Many people who use coaching are already motivated to change.**

- **A wellness coach is a particular kind of coach who supports clients to make positive choices around their fitness, nutrition, weight management, health risks and stress management.**

To become your own wellness coach you must learn to counter the inner anti-coach, take control of your choices and support yourself.

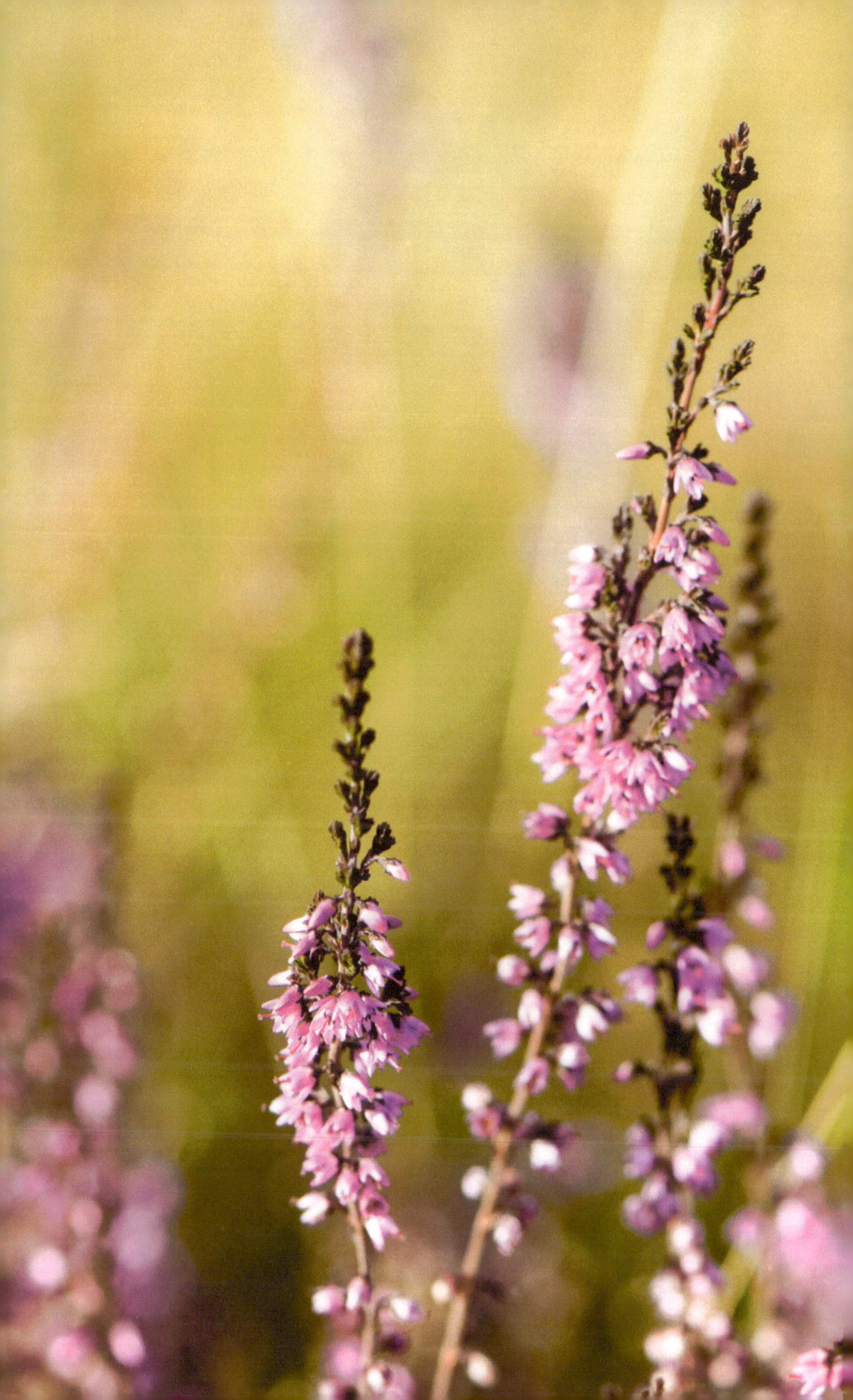

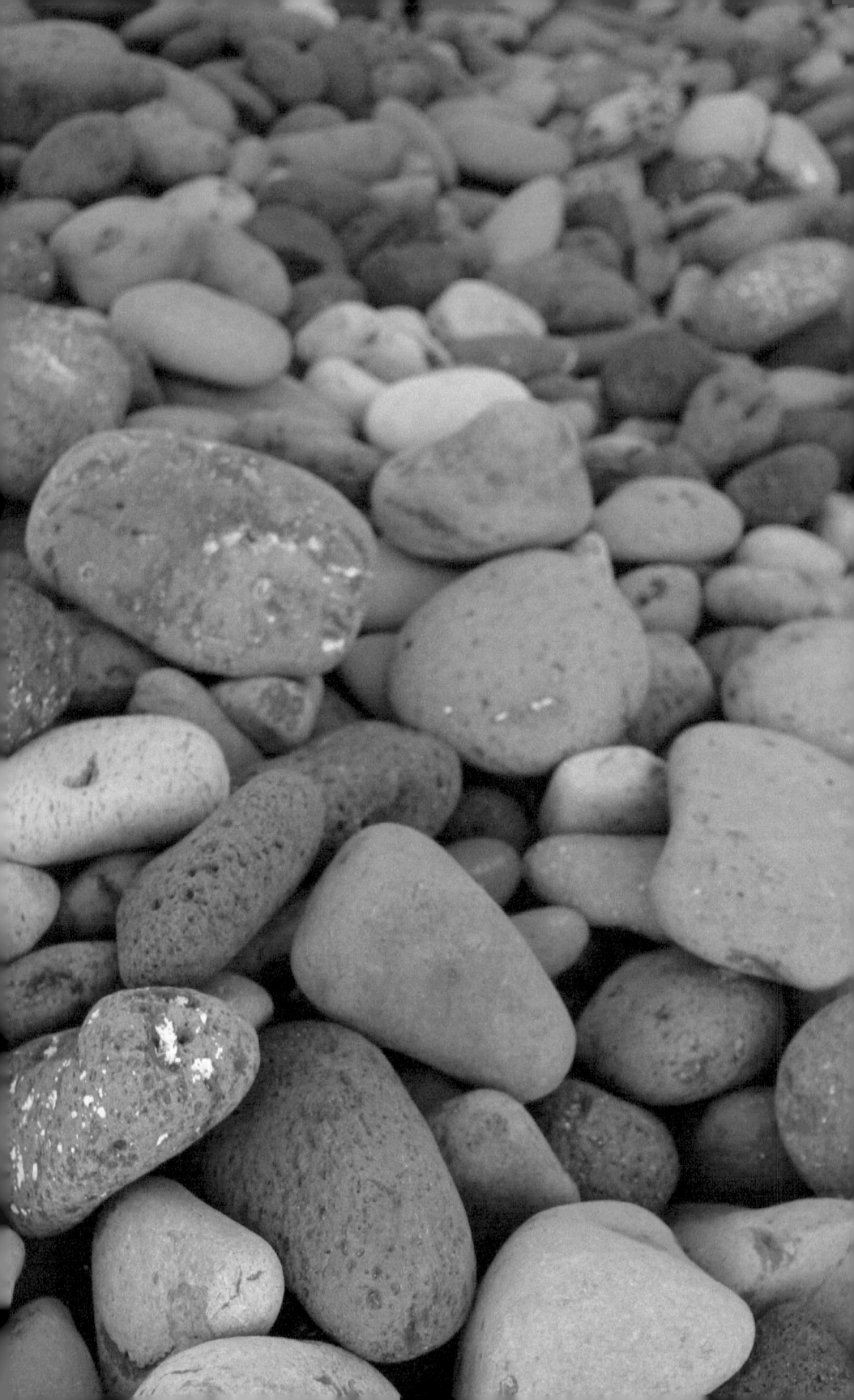

Section two

CREATING A VISION

What is your vision?

A vision is essentially a picture in our minds that can be described in words. It is clear, precise, colourful and real.

A wellness vision is a picture that focuses on health and vitality. It evokes feelings and a sense of movement. It can mobilise motivation, excitement and satisfaction.

Your wellness vision is a picture of the way you see yourself living when you have put into practice healthy behaviours that will achieve your goals. It will also have elements of other outcomes, usually the reasons you want to be well.

Your vision should be very real to you. It is what will keep you on track when the going gets tough.

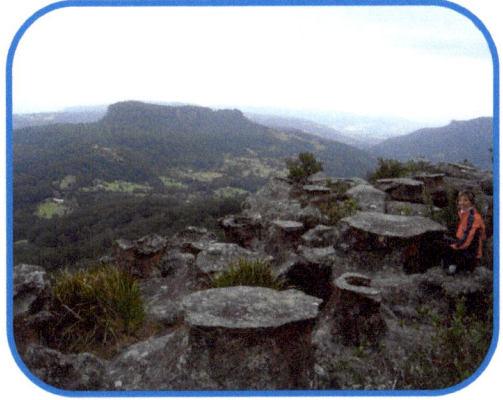

My wellness vision has changed over the years. When I was in my twenties, it was all about being the best I could be – more in terms of achievement and success. I was determined to run a marathon. I did, and the glory was shortlived but the sense of accomplishment stayed with me and helped build my confidence around other life goals. When I had children, my vision was more around staying well for them – to give them the best care I could, whilst still maintaining a sense of individuality. I'd given up my body to the reproduction process with a sense of awe. Once I got it back I was determined to make it "mine" again! Now the children are grown, my wellness vision has expanded yet again but with a subtle difference. I no longer want to push myself past certain limits; I want to keep my body and mind as well as they can be so I can get the most out of every moment in life. My wellness is my investment in my future. I so often see people who are tremendously successful in some areas of their life, but physically they are held back – dragging the chain so to speak. And I want them to feel how good it can be to be at their best in all areas of their lives. This is why I love what I do!

Fiona Cosgrove

What does your vision represent?

Your vision will reveal a way of living that you want to achieve. It will become the personal interpretation of health standards you wish to set for yourself. You will get a sense of how it would feel if you were fueling your body with good nutrition, and how much more energy you could have if you changed your exercise habits. This vision will give you a direction and a focus for what your life can be like. Your vision will be a picture of the best you can be.

Why do you want it?

This is the most important question you will ask yourself. If your vision includes living in a particular way, ask yourself, "Why does that matter to me?" The answer to this question says something about your values. It will provide the motivation to stay on track.

Sometimes the healthy behaviours become the vision itself. So our desire to stay fit and strong, for example, may be about ensuring that we can continue to enjoy our recreational passion.

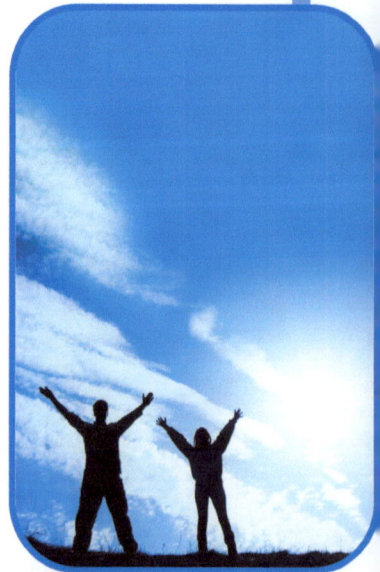

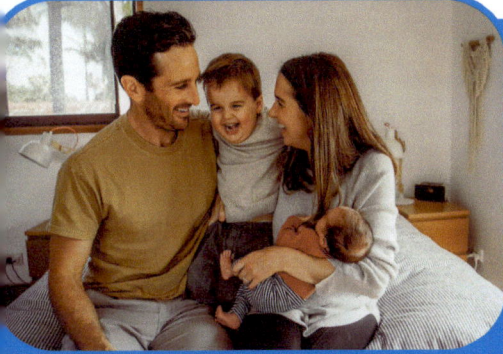

Prior to having kids I was into competitive sports including triathlon and running which I loved! I enjoyed being involved in these sports for physical and mental wellbeing. I was 'fit' and had a lot of time to myself to train. Since having kids my priorities have shifted and although my health and wellness is as ever as important, my time is scarce and precious. Health and wellness to me now is making sure I am physically and mentally well to care for my children and also to show them a good example of what being healthy is. Often when we have kids our wellbeing gets pushed to the bottom of the priorities and it's easy to get complacent. However, I have learnt quickly that if I carve out time for me and my wellness, I will always have the energy and health to be there for my family.

Kendyl Emoforpoulos

"I am determined to stay as fit, strong and mobile as long as possible with my limitations, so that I can continue to catch a wave any way I can."

Doug Iredale, former national surfing champion, after having a knee replacement and several reconstructions

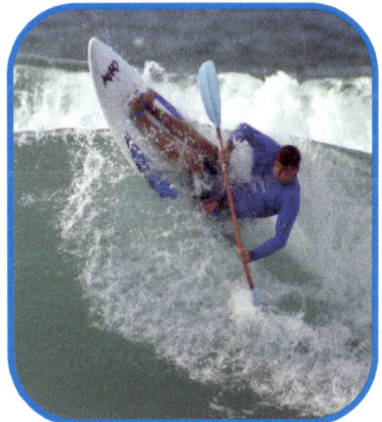

What are your strengths?

We all have unique abilities and strengths. Often they have been built in the face of adversity. These are resources we can tap into to help us achieve our goals. Generally, we are not very good at identifying them. Before you begin to set any goals, take some time to list at least five qualities you have that will help you. If you are struggling to think of them, look back on your life and remember any other times when you have accomplished something and what that took.

My strengths are:

1. Organised
2. Resilient
3. Determined
4. ?
5. ?
6. ?
7. ?

"I was always looking outside myself for strength and confidence but it comes from within. It is there all the time."

Anna Freud

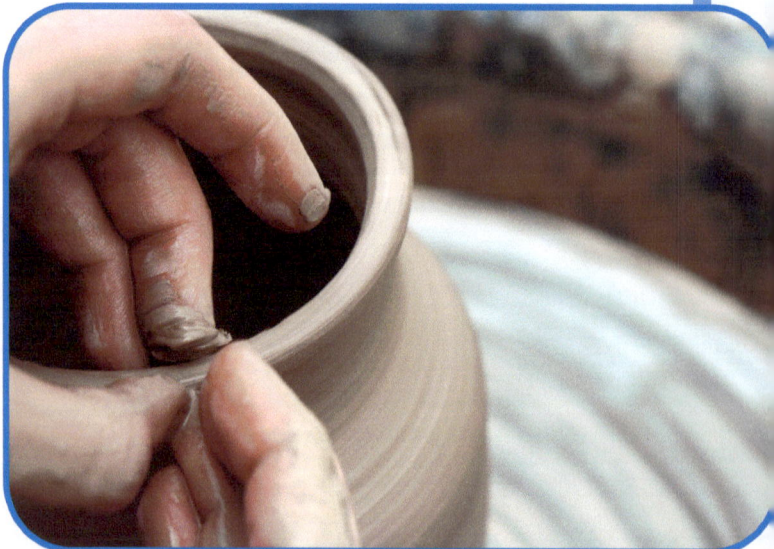

I want to lose weight but I don't think I have what it takes to change my bad eating habits – I love high-fat snacks!

… but I did give up smoking 10 years ago. That wasn't easy but I succeeded.

I want to exercise regularly but I don't know how I'll fit t in, I'm so pressed for time

…but I am very organised. I fit lots of things into my life and my secretary never lets me miss a work commitment.

What could get in the way?

Identifying the obstacles tends to be the easy part. We can usually come up with many things that will get in the way, the greatest one of which is frequently ourselves. We get in our own way.

Common obstacles include:

- Lack of time
- Competing priorities
- Dislike of exercise
- Hate running
- Other people
- Eating out
- No time to make healthy meals
- Travelling for work

All of these can be real obstacles. Sometimes they are harder to overcome than other factors which may fall into the "excuses" category. Recognising and naming them is the first step to overcoming them. Make your list and rank each obstacle 1, 2 or 3 – where 1 is a major hurdle and 3 is something that can fairly easily be negotiated; 2 is somewhere in the middle.

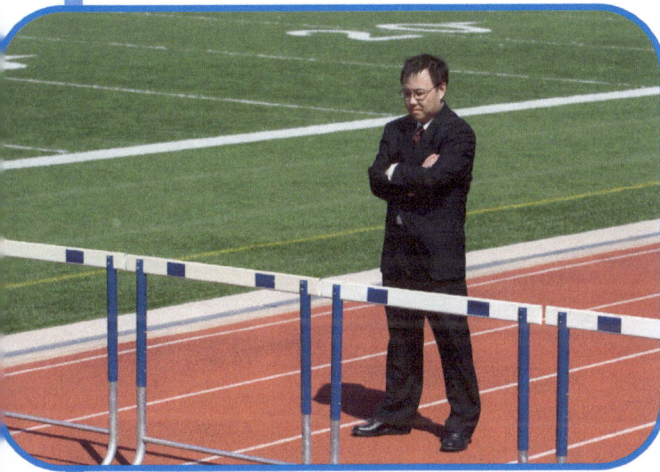

"Flow around obstacles, don't confront them, don't struggle to succeed. Wait for the right moment."

Lao Tzu

The next step is to roll up our sleeves and come up with some ideas to get past those obstacles.

"Challenges can be stepping stones or stumbling blocks. It's just a matter of how you view them."

Author unidentified.

What are some possible strategies?

This is a time to be creative. Don't rule out any possibility. List all ideas then pick out the ones that you like the sound of and that seem manageable. This is your first lesson in problem-solving. Enlist someone's support if necessary. Take time with this exercise; it is one of the most important.

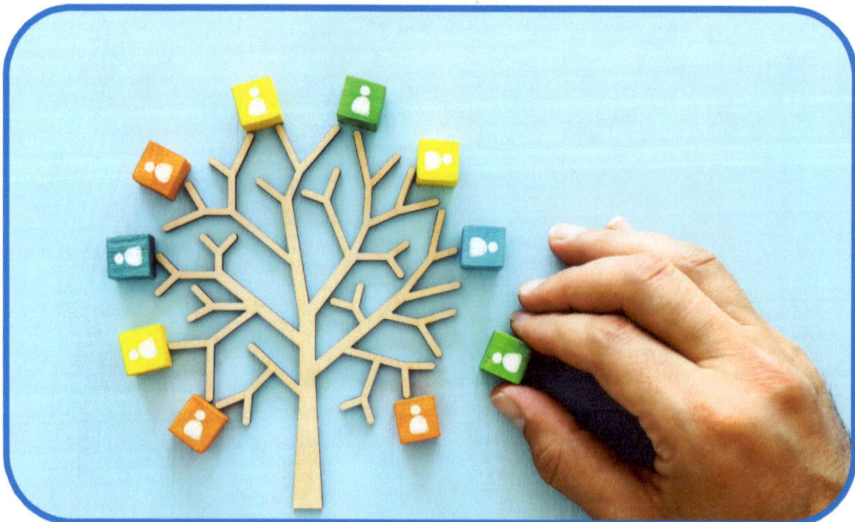

Obstacle: Lack of time
- Go to bed earlier so can get up earlier
- Leave work at 6pm
- Work smarter, not harder
- Analyse working day
- Delegate some tasks or duties
- Ask for help from family or friends
- Employ someone to ease workload

Obstacle: Hate running
- Start with walking, increase pace, try run/walking

Obstacle: Lack of time to make healthy meals
- Prepare at weekend and freeze
- Find new recipes in quick and healthy cook books

Obstacle: Travel interferes with exercise program
- Get a trainer to write a portable program
- Buy a band and do resistance work
- Only stay in hotels with gyms

If you got it, what else would change?

Changing our lifestyle to produce better health and wellness can have an interesting side effect. In order to change our habits, we have to increase our awareness. One of the features of a habit is that it requires little thought. Generally, we're on auto-pilot when acting out a habit, and therefore we do it without really thinking about what we are doing and what it might mean to us in terms of consequences. When our awareness is heightened in one area of our "living" routine, it can suddenly turn the spotlight on other areas and the flow-on from that can be tremendous.

This can happen in two ways:

Firstly, the sense of confidence that you get from making successful change by setting goals and achieving them can lead you to consider changing something else in your life that, up until now, had seemed too daunting to tackle. The belief that you can master one area of your life can help you move mountains in others.

The second element in this scenario is that suddenly things that previously had seemed tolerable now become highlighted. The need to make further changes gets moved forward in importance.

> **Possibilities**
>
> If I could get my weight under control I might then have the confidence to go for a promotion.

"We first make our habits and then our habits make us."

Anonymous

Tolerations

What am I putting up with in my life?

1. My job
2. My poor fitness
3. My weight

What is this costing me?

- Lost years of my life feeling dulled
- Hours in the day when I could have more energy
- Not feeling good about myself

How can I change this?

- Start to think about a career change
- Start an exercise program
- Change my eating plan

"I had a friend who was on such an emotional high after completing his first marathon that he decided there was nothing in life he couldn't achieve. He resigned from his job, set up a small business, wrote six books and now is worth millions."
Dr. John Lang

"A moment's insight is sometimes worth a life's experience."

Oliver Wendell Holmes

Summary

In this section, we have explored the following questions:

- **Who would you be if you were at your best?**

- **How big is the gap between where you are now and where you would like to be?**

- **What are your deepest reasons for wanting those changes?**

- **What are the personal strengths that could help you with your plan?**

- **What have you achieved in the past that took effort?**

- **What could get in the way of your plan to change?**

- **Are they real obstacles or ones that can easily be overcome?**

- **What are some strategies for getting past the obstacles?**

- **What, if anything, could also change if you were successful in this area of your life?**

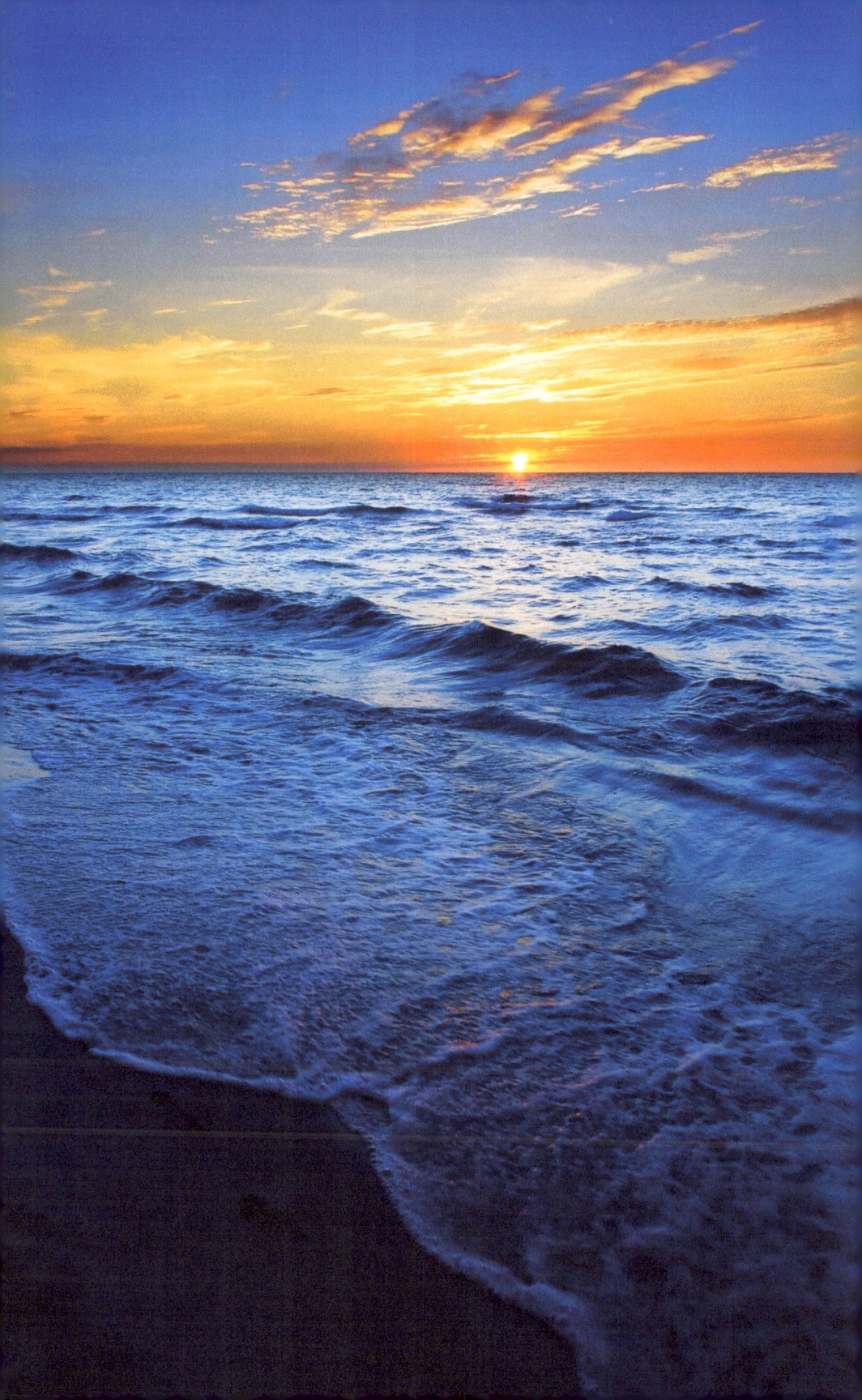

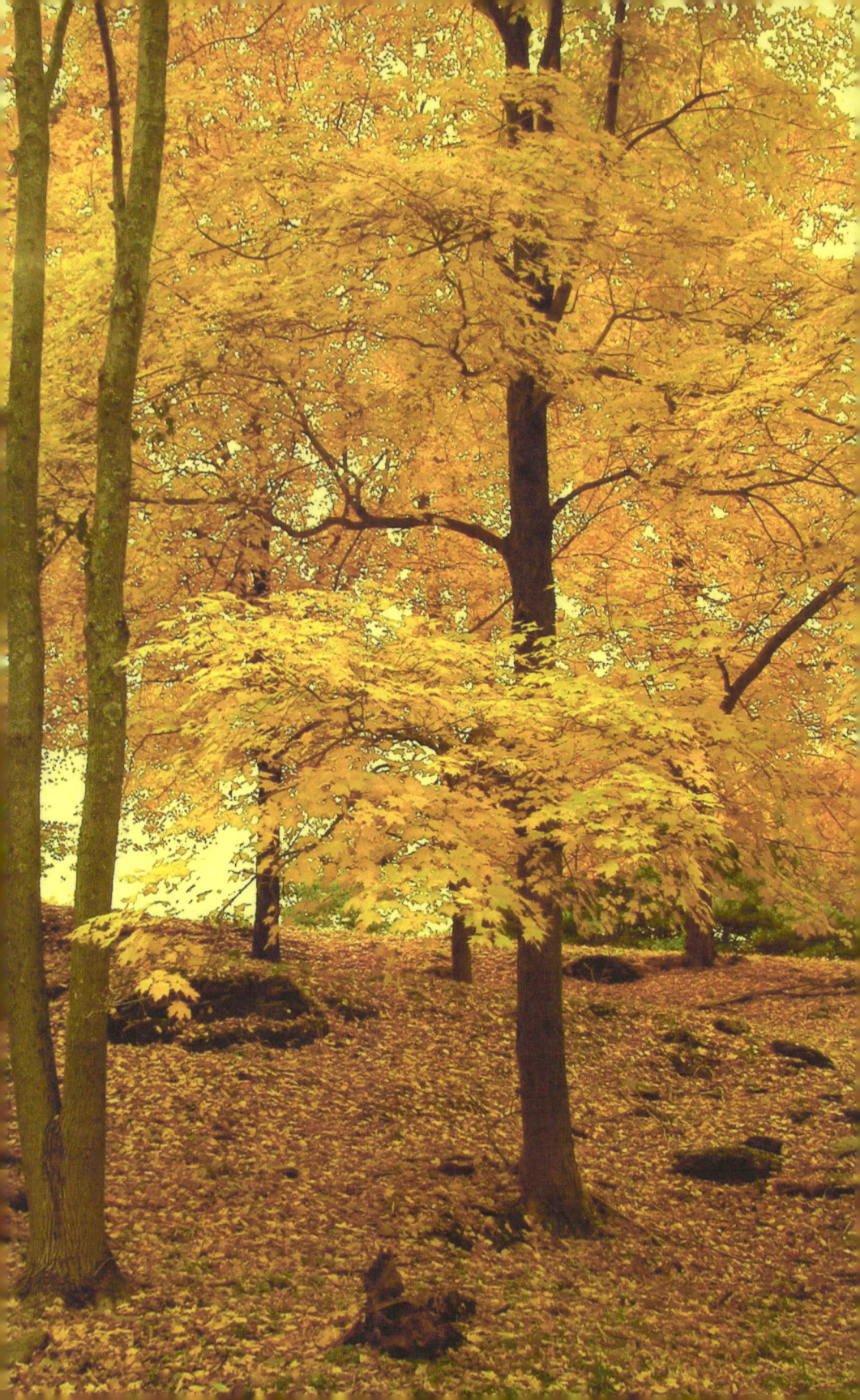

Section three

CHANGING
BEHAVIOUR

Change – how can we create it?

Changing behaviour can be very simple or very complex. Much of our life is made up of habits – some are more ingrained than others, and some give us more satisfaction or gratification than others. If you want to stop losing your keys, for example, it may only take 21 days of putting them in a designated spot at home for this to become the new habit. Problem solved.

If, however, we want to change the habit of being inactive for many years, then this needs approaching in a different way. Getting out of bed and walking each morning for 21 days would be a similar approach to the problem above. But for most people, there is a great deal of missing work that has to be done to make this happen. We want the change to last beyond the 21 days.

There are many factors that influence our success at changing behaviour. As you will see in coming sections, there are many building blocks to change. And most of these require "thinking" work rather than "doing" work. This can be quite challenging for those of us who like ACTION. We want it and we want it now!

The truth is, if the thinking work is not done, then change runs the risk of only ever being a flash in the pan. So before we get started on climbing the mountain to lasting change, it is

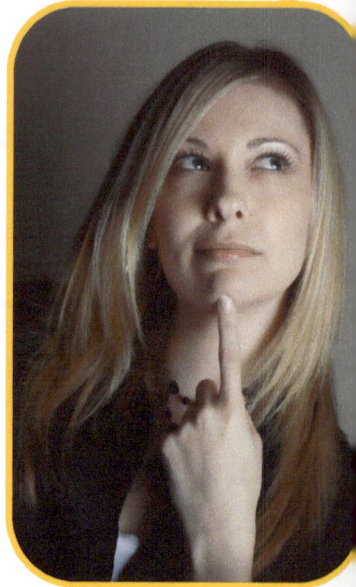

worth considering some of the following things that might trip you up, or at least influence your thinking process.

The role of motivation

"I am just not motivated" is a common complaint. So where does motivation come from and what exactly is it?

Motivation is impacted by a range of internal and external sources. It comes from our values, from our self-esteem and self-image, from our field of expectations around what is possible for us and from life-long messages we have internalised about ourselves.

Essentially, these things determine the way we perceive cost versus benefit in our behaviours, decisions and goals. When we have decided to make a change, it is usually the result of having come to a realisation that the cost of the current behaviour is outweighing any benefits. A big part of motivation comes from acknowledging we are in some kind of pain or discomfort and it is no longer worth it.

Motivation is also a process. There will be times when you have less willingness to do what you have to do to create change. This is why it is important to have many strategies or tools in your tool box, to fall back on when motivation is low.

The role of fear

When considering change, people are often fearful for different reasons. Fear can work for or against change. Consider the following:

Fear that keeps us stuck

1. Fear of failure

How many things have we not done because we were secretly afraid of failing? Why is failure so scary? We are worried that others will think less of us and also that we will think less of ourselves – lowered self-esteem. The reality is that without failure, or mistakes, _we can never learn anything_. We should be looking for opportunities to try new challenges, not to show we can always succeed but to build strength and resilience in the face of defeat or setback and a chance to grow and learn From our mistakes.

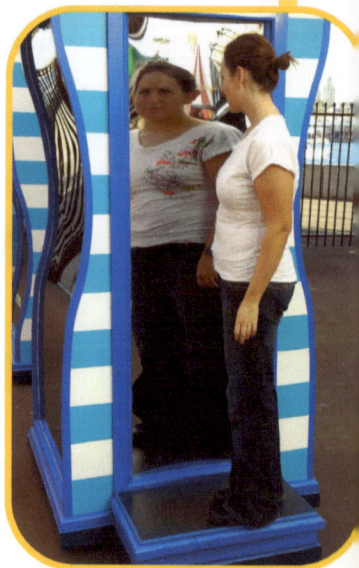

"The greatest mistake you can make in life is to continually fear you will make one."

Elbert Hubbard

2. Fear of not being able to adapt to the outcome of change

So what if I do manage to lose weight? Or get fitter? My life will change in many ways and even my identity could be different. Is this something I can cope with? I may have to buy new clothes or even face new situations when people see me in a different way. This means stepping out of my comfort zones. We often forget to visualise all the outcomes of achieving our goals. That is what our vision is for – to remind us.

3. Fear of not being accepted by others or losing love of others

We have often been doing things a certain way for a long time. Introducing new healthy behaviours can influence many facets of our life, particularly when it comes to relationships and our social support structures. When we adopt a healthier lifestyle, this can be confronting for some people in our lives. Their expectations of us may no longer be met as we take on different roles and ways of being. Our healthy changes also have the effect of highlighting other people's not so healthy choices, and this can be confronting. Sometimes, a change in our social activities and groups of friends is necessary. The flip side is to remember how good it can be to be a role model for the people we love.

These three fears can keep us stuck, but fear can also push us forward.

Snapshot – Not Fat John anymore

"When I lost a lot of weight, the world opened up to me in ways I hadn't expected. At times, it was confronting as I had to deal with new experiences and people sometimes seemed uncomfortable because they weren't talking to 'Fat John'. It was like taking on a new identity. But I love who I am now."

If I make this change...

What else could change?

Why does that worry me?

"Fear will never go away as long as we continue to grow."

Susan Jeffers

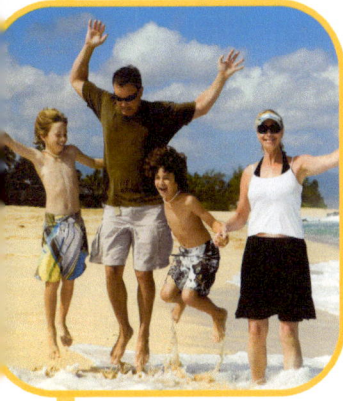

Fear that helps us move

Fear of harm to ourselves by continuing to live an unhealthy lifestyle

If we have a good sense of caring for ourselves, we can use this to help move us forward. Who wants to die young or develop one of the many lifestyle-related illnesses that abound?

A precipitating event can promote change through fear

There are times when something happens that can cause sudden and dramatic fear for our health. Death or illness of a close friend or family member; medical test results that reveal a hidden condition; even falling in love or having a child can change our outlook on how healthy we wish to be. This fear can be used in a positive way.

Life will always have an element of fear.

The role of ambivalence

Part of the complexity of being human is our ability to see ourselves in different situations so that we can make choices based on what we think would be a good move. Whilst we can imagine what it would be like to be fit, vital and in good health, we can also imagine the sense of loss that might result from giving up our current, comfortable existence. There may also be doubt about success (fear) and some anxiety about what else would change in our lives. On the one hand, we want to improve our wellness; on the other, we want to preserve the status quo. After all, if there wasn't some benefit to the status quo, we would have changed it already.

One way of working through this is to create a list of advantages and disadvantages of both states – being well and being not so well. For example remaining overweight or losing weight, staying unfit or getting fitter, giving up smoking or continuing to smoke. We call this Decisional Balance. When the list of pros for changing becomes longer than the list of cons, then you are ready to prepare to take action. If it's the other way round, more work needs to be done before you begin. Exploring ambivalence is the key to uncovering motivation for change.

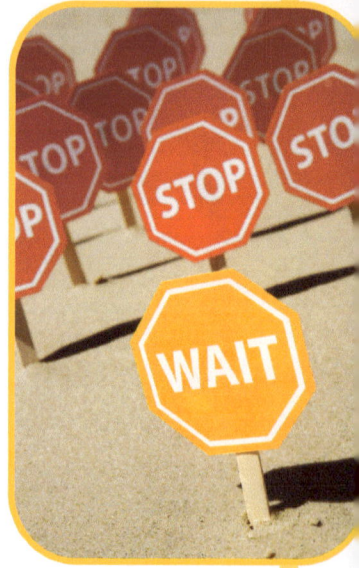

The role of love

The opposite of fear is love. When we consider improving our health and wellness, this can be relevant in two ways.

Firstly, love for ourselves can motivate us to make the change. Self-care is one way of putting it; self-esteem is another. Because taking positive action to become better is self-caring behaviour, it can't help but increase our self-esteem. If we can't care for ourselves, how can we care for the others that we love?

This brings us to the second way love can move us to change. The realisation that we love our family and that we matter to them can prompt a new appreciation of our value. While people depend on and care about us, it makes sense to lead a healthy lifestyle. Other people need us to look after ourselves – and they know we're worth it. Maybe they have a point?

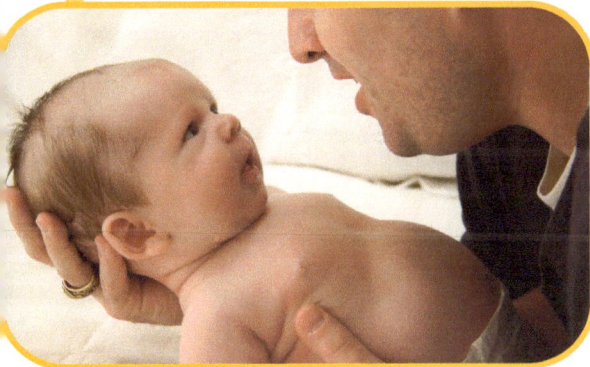

"Each of us must be willing to stand out while fitting into society."

Denis Waitley, 1995

The role of society – what messages do we receive each day?

Society will affect our actions in two ways. Depending on the culture of the organisation you work in, the town you live in, the family you come from, and the country you inhabit, your views about wellness will differ.

If everyone around you eats a diet high in saturated fat and takeaway food, this will seem like the norm. It will be much harder to change when you are the only one stepping out of line. If everyone in your household hates exercise, you will have a harder time beginning to be active.

But it can be done. You can even become a catalyst for change in the lives of others.

Meanwhile, you are likely to also be noticing more messages in the media about the high incidence of obesity, the need for regular activity and the risks of living a highly stressed life. These messages are also affecting your attitudes towards changing your habits.

This effect is known as "consciousness raising" and is very important for people who are in the pre-contemplation and contemplation stages of change, as it can provide the impetus to move to the next stage. Fortunately, society is starting to take notice of how our busy lifestyles, addictions and fast-food diets are taking a toll on the health of the nation.

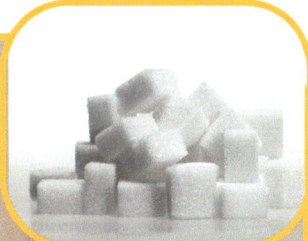

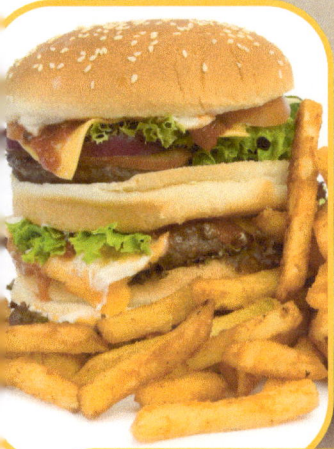

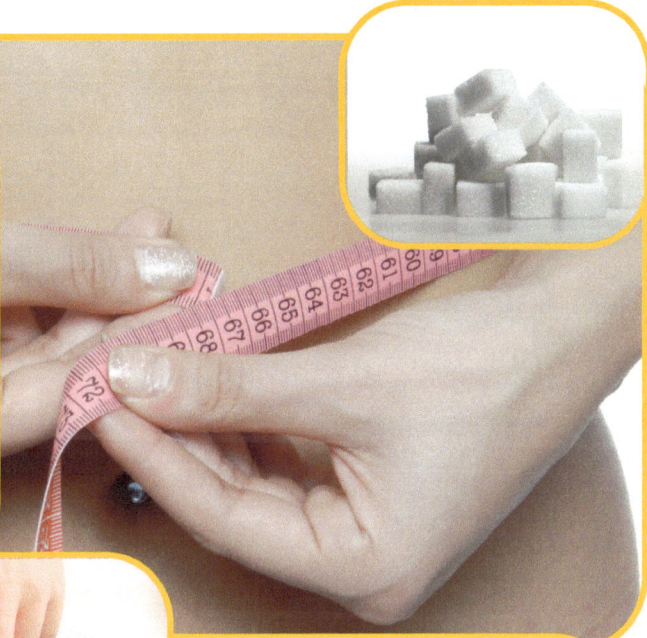

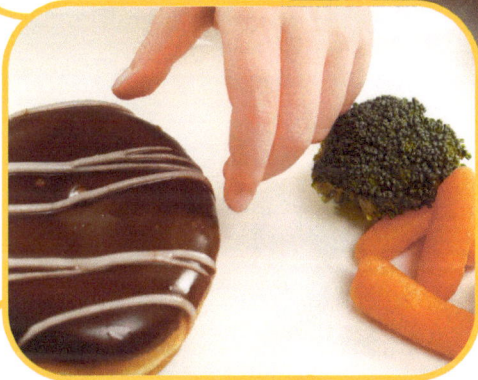

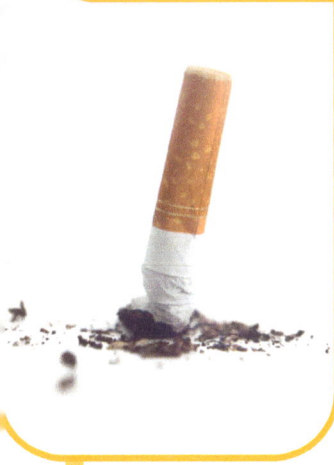

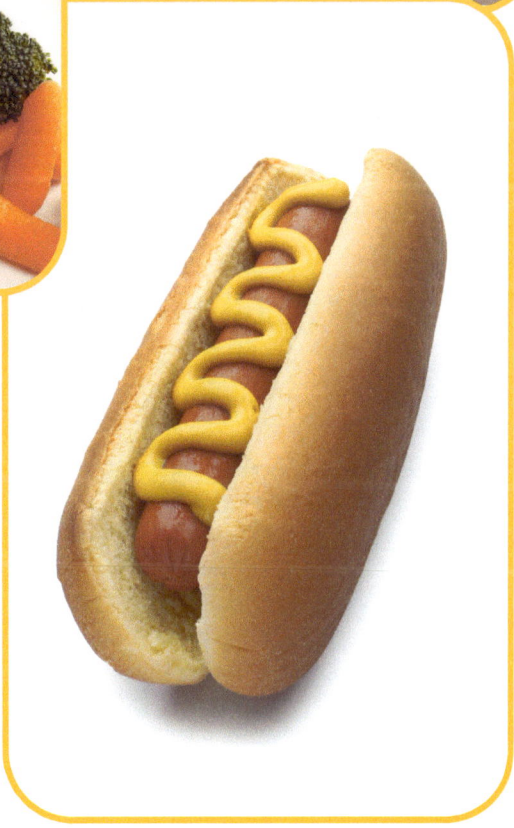

Understanding the stages of change

Research has shown that when it comes to change, we all fall into one of six categories at any given point in time, for any given behaviour that we choose to engage in.

We can move backwards and forwards through the stages but by answering a simple question, we can determine what stage we are at. The stages are classified as:

- Pre-contemplation
  I won't or I can't

- Contemplation
  I may

- Preparation
  I will

- Action
  I am

- Maintenance
  I still am

- Relapse
  I was

STAGES OF CHANGE

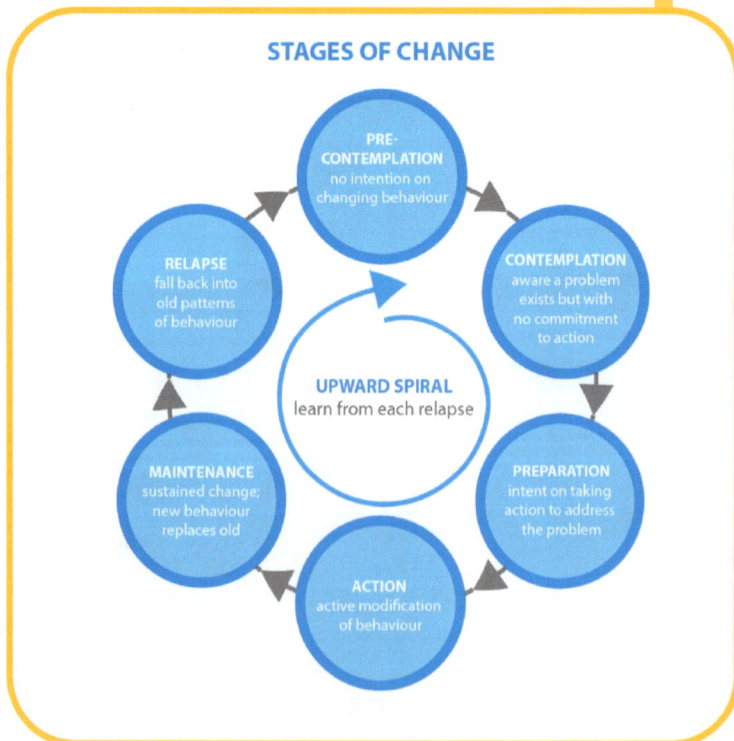

PRE-CONTEMPLATION
no intention on changing behaviour

CONTEMPLATION
aware a problem exists but with no commitment to action

PREPARATION
intent on taking action to address the problem

ACTION
active modification of behaviour

MAINTENANCE
sustained change; new behaviour replaces old

RELAPSE
fall back into old patterns of behaviour

UPWARD SPIRAL
learn from each relapse

Prochaska, J., Norcross, J. and Diclemente, C. (1994; 2002) *Changing for Good.*

The questions to ask are:

Pre-contemplation: Are you thinking of making a change?

Contemplation: Are you thinking of making a change in the next six months?

Preparation: Have you taken initial steps towards making a change and are you getting ready to implement the change in the next month?

Action: Have you begun the new behaviour?

Maintenance: Are you regularly performing the new behaviour?

Relapse: Have you stopped the new behaviour and slipped back into old patterns?

Prochaska, J., Norcross, J. and Diclemente, C. (1994; 2002) *Changing for Good.*

Why do we often fail in our attempts to improve our lifestyle?

There are many reasons for falling by the wayside. The main one seems to be that we are not ready to take action. The stages of change model illustrates how we need to move through several stages before we begin. The importance of this varies according to the type of change you want to make. Some behaviours take more preparation than others, for example changing your diet needs some planning, as does starting an exercise program. Giving up smoking can be done suddenly but the "cold turkey" approach doesn't always work for everyone and people begin to think of themselves as "serial quitters".

"I am a serial gym joiner. I join, I drop out, I join another gym, I drop out."

What chance of success do you think this person has when these are her comments upon enquiring about membership at a health club?

Not high, right? So in order to increase our chances of success, we need to be fully prepared to make the change. And that includes many things we have discussed already, like:

- Creating a vision

- Working out strategies

What can help you move to the next stage? ...

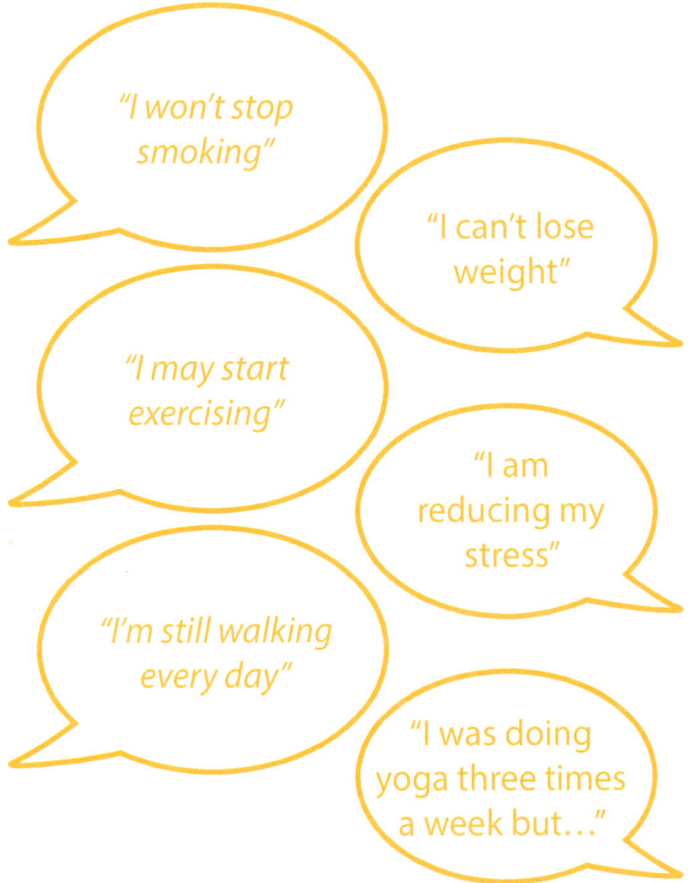

"I won't stop smoking"

"I can't lose weight"

"I may start exercising"

"I am reducing my stress"

"I'm still walking every day"

"I was doing yoga three times a week but…"

Pre-empting obstacles and planning how to overcome them

- Enlisting the support of others
- Recognising our strengths
- Increasing our belief that we can do it

This takes time and preparation. And it will pay off.

Which stage are you at?

By now you probably have a good idea of which stage you are at with regard to the different changes that are possible in your wellness. Keep referring back to your vision to remember why you wish to make any change and what will be at the end of it.

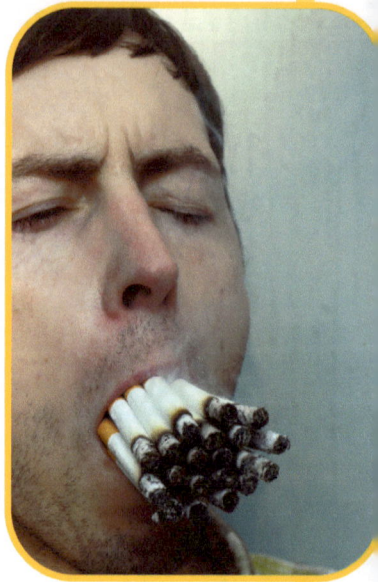

There are certain processes that can help you along the way and these are described below.

So, take out your wellness journal and note where you are at for each desired behaviour change.

Are you saying:

I won't or I can't

I may

I will

I am

I still am

I was

…In the pre-contemplation and contemplation stages

Becoming more aware of what your current habits are costing you (Consciousness raising)

- Exploring the advantages of change can be helpful, including getting scientific information about the risks of not changing.

- Looking at family history and assessing risk can be useful.

- If you are an "I won't" person, carefully consider pros for change and see how they might fit into your vision.

- Understand that if you are contemplating change, you are likely to have ambivalence and lack of confidence around success. This is normal.

- As discussed earlier, you may have some anxiety about what life will be like when you are successful. Don't ignore this feeling. It is also normal.

Giving up smoking - Stage - Contemplation What can help?

- Reading literature about what smoking does to your body.

- Someone telling you that your breath smells.

- A friend leaving the room when you light up.

Feeling the discomfort and excitement about possible movement towards your vision (Emotional arousal)

- This is where you can focus clearly on the advantages that fit well with your vision and your values. A careful analysis of the things that could make it difficult and strategies to overcome them is essential.

- Thinking of where you could start and how you could break the behaviour change into small and easy steps will also help.

Self re-evaluation

- Reviewing your strengths and the successes you have had in the past can feed your confidence to go on.

- Who do you want to be that you're not being now?

- Are you happy with where you are and does it fit with your values?

...In the preparation stage

You have made up your mind. You may even have begun new behaviours or at least the groundwork to adopt them. Any information that helps you know what to do and how the new behaviour should look will be of use now.

Changing my eating habits to enable me to lose weight – Stage - Preparation

What can help?

- Identifying strategies in other people's success stories.

- Finding out about eating plans.

- Keeping a record of what you are eating – a food diary.

USEFUL INFORMATION
Weight loss is in the head

A project called National Weight Control Registry (NWCR) was created in 1993 to study the differences between people who lose weight and maintain the weight loss, and those who put it back on again (95% of dieters). Results have shown that the people who kept the weight off have a tendency to process information with the part of their brain that is very methodical, disciplined, structured, punctual and neat which makes it easier for them to stick to a routine and the sometimes laborious process of following a diet. (We can train ourselves to do this, by the way).

Herrmann International developed the Herrmann Brain Dominance Instrument (HBDI) to assess people's thinking styles. They now recommend activities that encourage systematic and detail-oriented methods of thinking. These include:

Organising and alphabetising certain possessions
– your CDs or spice drawer.

Keeping a log of daily activities.

Planning your week.

Sorting out your closet.

Following a recipe, step by step.

Try and make the activities as appealing as you can to your natural thinking or processing style. For example, involve other people if this makes it easier. Dream and plan for something more abstract. This preparation will help when it comes to the work involved in maintaining a new eating plan.

Making a commitment (Self-liberation)

Decide to do it. Write it down and tell someone.

The act of committing your plan to paper is a way of making it exist outside your head. You can even sign it as a contract with yourself. It can also really help to say it out loud and have your declaration heard and witnessed by others. Not only does this help keep you accountable, it gives you someone with whom to celebrate your decision to change.

Enlisting support (Helping relationships)

Now it's time to make your plan concrete. Decide which club to join, whether to use a personal trainer, which training buddy to enlist, which foods to eliminate and what to substitute them with.

Having shared your commitment to change with others, identify ways they can support you and ask them for specific behaviours that will help you. Enlisting the support of others can be particularly worthwhile around anything you can identify that might get in the way of change.

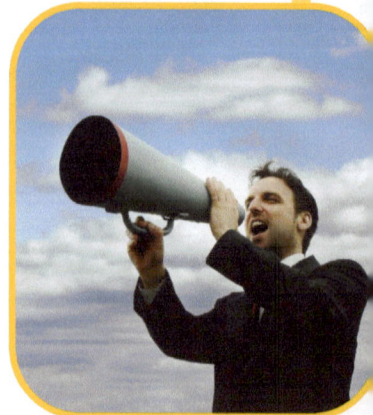

...When action has begun

Substitute alternative behaviour (Counter conditioning)

Now you are doing something to change. What is the new behaviour? Instead of thinking of taking something out of your life, think of how you can put something new into it.

What is going to get in the way? (Contingency management)

It is inevitable that things will come up to make your new way of living difficult. Every time you set a goal for the week, think what could get in the way and come up with one or two strategies to overcome that. E.g. instead of going out for a drink on Friday after work, you make a plan to do an exercise class with a friend.

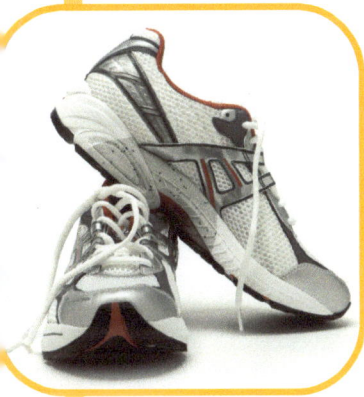

Creating cues (Stimulus/ environment control)

We are creatures of habit and association. It's amazing what impact a new pair of running shoes can have on our attitude to getting out there; or a new gym bag; or finding an organic food shop. Try some of these simple ideas:

- Keep a fresh set of exercise gear in your car.

- Hang the pair of pants you wish to fit into in your room, in full view.

- Create a fruit bowl full of colourful choices and keep it stocked – on your desk.

- Have bottles of sparkling water in the fridge.

- Display photos of how you would like to look - or not look!

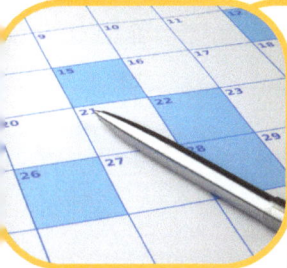

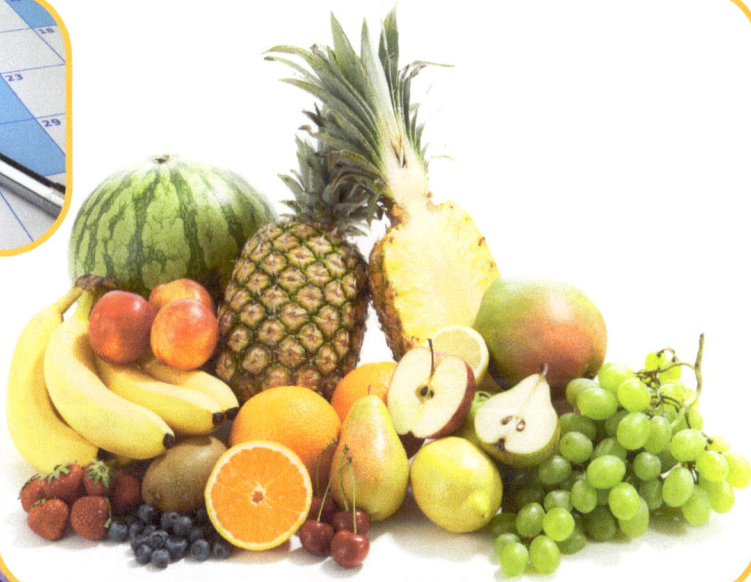

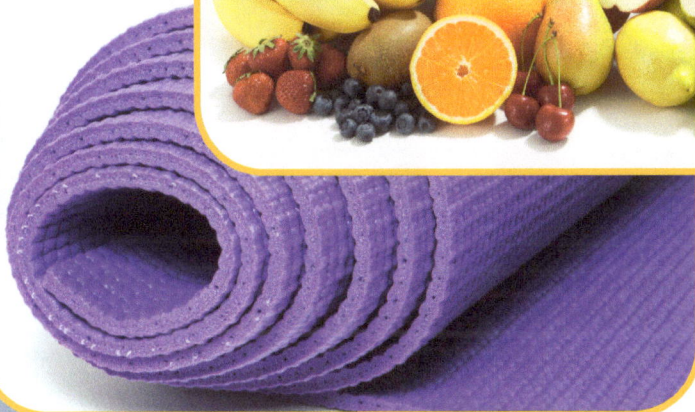

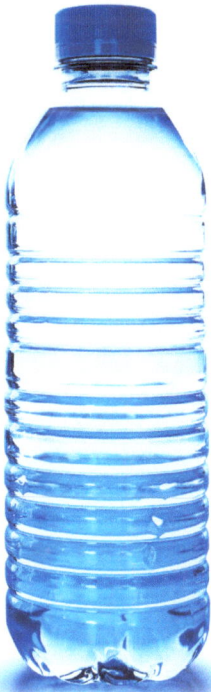

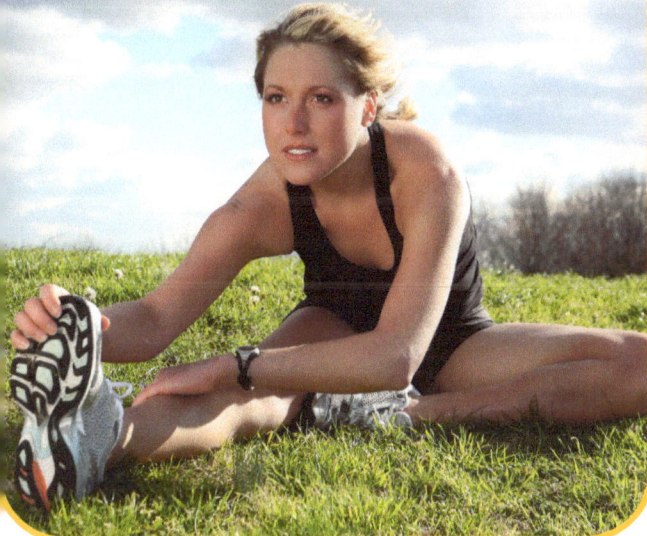

Summary

- Changing behaviour is essentially a bout changing habits.

- Motivation is a fluctuating factor which cannot be relied on to sustain the path to lasting change.

- Fear can play a part – fear of failure, fear of adapting, fear of not being accepted and fear of harming ourselves or loved ones can all make us move in the direction of positive change.

- Ambivalence is normal and creating a decisional balance sheet can help.

- Nurturing a healthy self-esteem is crucial and love for others can support our efforts.

- Society influences us in different ways. The culture of our environments – our workplace, our family and our society - will affect our choices.

- We are all at a certain stage of change for each set of behaviours in which we engage. Identifying the stage will help us know what will move us forward.

- Preparation is essential before any change plan can be successful.

- There are certain processes that can help at each stage of change.

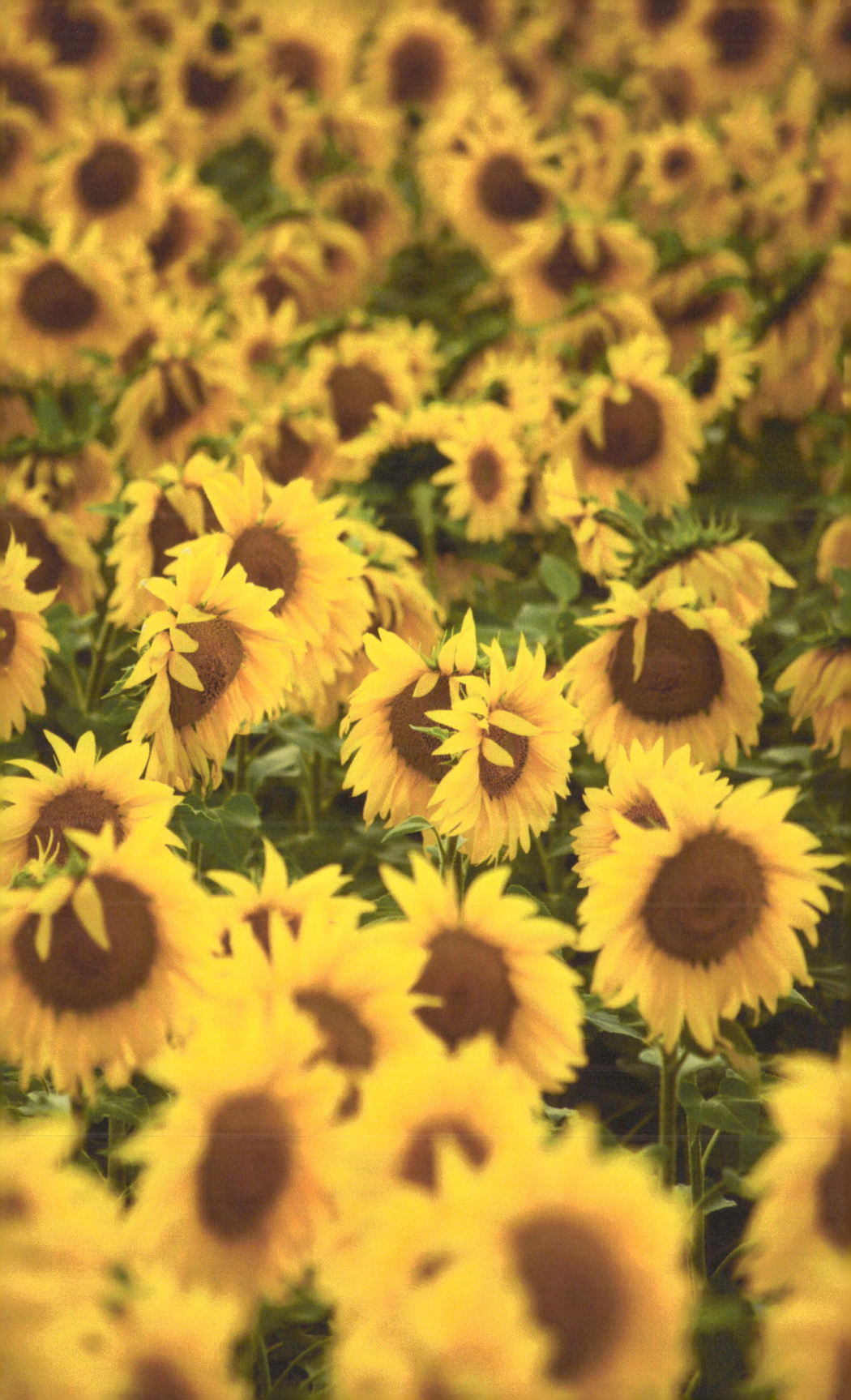

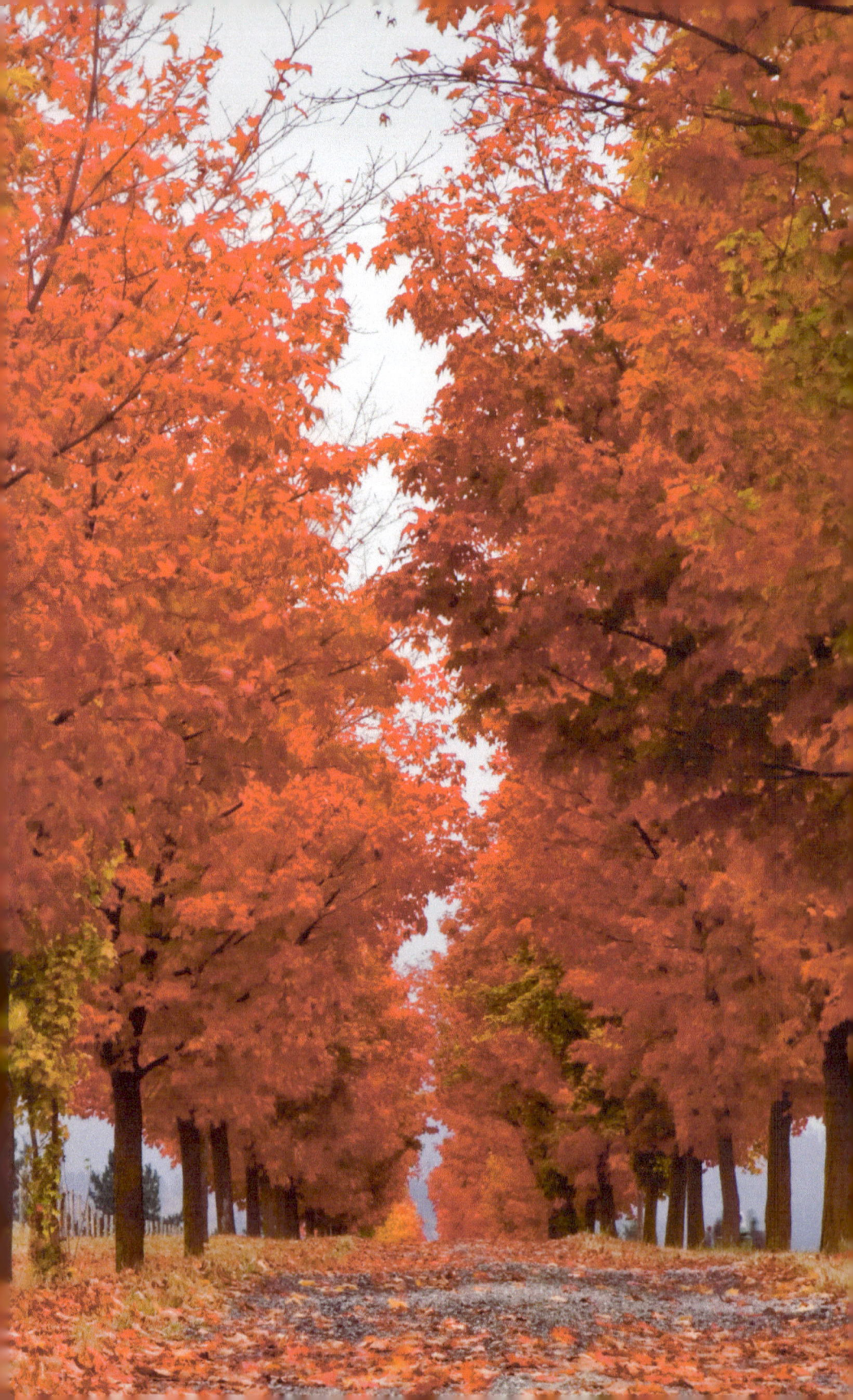

Section four

THE JOURNEY

Climbing Mount Lasting Change

Now you understand the stages of change and you have a clearer idea of which stage you are at for each area of your wellness. The next step is exploring how we build a strong foundation to make change (new behaviour) stick.

Think of change as being like a hill, or a pyramid, that needs to be built, then climbed - call it "Mount Lasting Change". At the pinnacle will be the person you truly want to be.

The following picture shows building blocks that help to create a strong foundation upon which to build lasting change and a new life. It's possible to leave one or two out, but the foundation will be stronger if all the building blocks are included.

It's important to remember that progress towards lasting change is rarely made on a continuous straight upwards path. We might climb one level then retrace our steps to do more work on the level below, then step up again, go sideways, forward, back and so on.

Mount Lasting Change

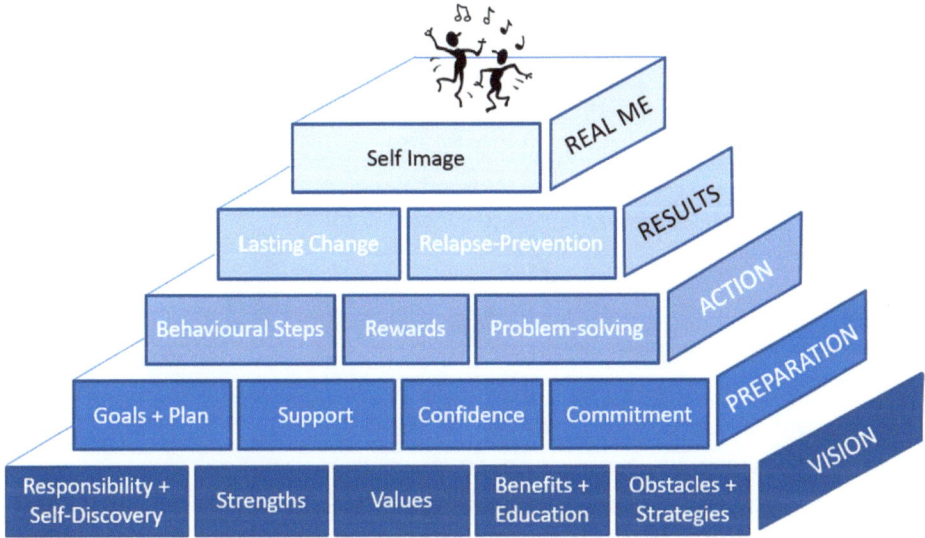

©This image is reproduced with the permission of Wellcoaches Corporation.

VISION

Let's look at the ground floor. There are five building blocks that really need to be put in place in order to lay the foundation for lasting change. Because we tend to be rather impatient about getting to the top, these building blocks are often overlooked. However, doing the groundwork is an essential part of bringing your vision to life and creating the conditions for the kind of change that is both meaningful and sustainable.

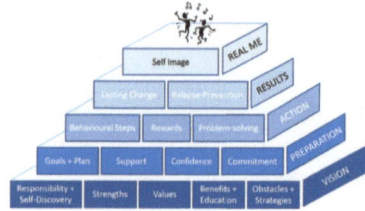

Responsibility and self-awareness

This is thinking work. In order to make behaviour change stick, you need to own the reasons you are making changes, and your power to make them. It is not about anyone else's agenda. It is not about blaming anyone, anything or any circumstances for your present situation. This building block will be created when you can make truthful and confident statements like:

"I want to lose weight and the only way that is going to happen is if I make it happen."

"I have become very unfit and I will change to become an active person again. The reasons for my lack of fitness are the choices I have made in recent months. I now choose to make better choices and realise that no one person can do this for me."

"My high levels of stress are undermining my enjoyment of life. I have allowed work pressure to affect my sleep and family life and I am now going to take steps to reduce my stress."

These statements are internal decisions with external declarations of what it will take to change. The key factor is that the responsibility lies with you - the person who wants to change. The very first step in any change is accepting that responsibility. A process of self-discovery can bring you to this realisation; a process that involves some committed reflection on what is not working for you and what you are willing to do about it.

"What am I tolerating in my health and wellness that is affecting the quality of my life?"

"What can I do to change this?"

You have brains in your head. You have feet in your shoes. You can steer yourself any direction you choose. You're on your own. And you know what you know. And YOU are the one who'll decide where to go!

Dr. Seuss

Strengths

Having given yourself a strong dose of reality, it's time to take stock of your assets. This is a process of recognising and honouring the qualities and resources you have that will help you succeed. It is easy to think of past failed attempts and label ourselves as "no good at sticking to an eating plan", or "someone who joins and drops out of health clubs". Instead, try thinking of things you have done in your life that have been successful. What qualities and resources were you able to draw on then? How might those assets of yours be invested in this new behaviour change?

"I am a very organised person."

"I gave up smoking some years ago."

"I studied for six years before I got my degree but I did get there."

"I am a very positive person who looks at mistakes as minor setbacks."

Identify your strengths, own them and enjoy the confidence that this acknowledgment will bring.

Values

This is an extremely important building block. You are only thinking of changing because the way you are living is in some way out of alignment with your beliefs. Explore the desired behaviour change and uncover what it is about your present situation that really irks you. Yes, it may be uncomfortable to carry extra kilos, but do you perhaps have a value around being active, or people looking their best, or being a good role model for younger people? If you look closely enough you will find the main reason for wanting to change. And this may be much deeper than you originally thought. Your values are what will help you work out the strongest motivating forces – because they represent what matters most to you.

When it comes to behaviour change, values are pure gold. They are the fuel that fires the engine and what helps you create your vision. As your values come to light, you may start to understand further reasons for change and want to slot these into your vision.

What is important to me in life? What do I value most?

(Remember that you will also place a value on existing habits that you want to change.)

What is important to me in the area of wellness?

Why is that important?

What is it costing me not to live by that value?

Benefits and education

This is the time when you find out what the adverse effects of not changing could be. What happens if you stay the same? These details will add substance to your vision and give you further reasons to act. Information may come in different forms. For example, a health check could reveal high blood pressure. A doctor might then explain what risks this carries. A smoker could become aware of how awful a death from lung cancer can be. New facts regarding the effects of daily drinking of alcohol could appear in the press. You may decide that a trek in Nepal is the best way of seeing the country and realise that with the right training this can become a reality. Watching a close friend start to look vital and younger from taking up yoga could strike a chord with you. This is the time you are creating your list of "pros" in the decisional balance. But there is an important distinction to make. Only the "pros" that you personally care about are important.

- What could I gain by changing?
- What do I stand to lose by not changing?

Obstacles and strategies

The obstacles that could get in the way may appear on your list of "cons". It's best to face them truthfully and see them as challenges rather than reasons not to change. Meeting the challenges and tackling the obstacles will be the source of your sense of mastery and achievement in the end. After all, there is no triumph without adversity.

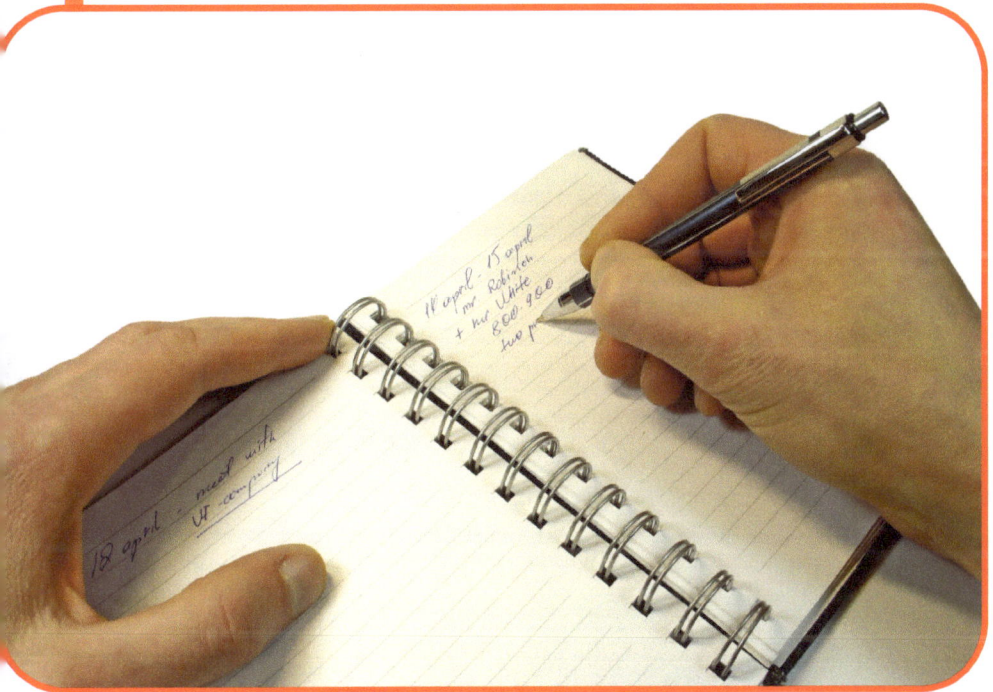

Obstacles come in two sizes. There are the big ones that need to be addressed before you begin. By airing and examining them you are facing the reality of what has got in the way in the past. For example, including exercise in your weekly schedule could be perceived as just another time pressure. "How can I possibly find time to exercise when I am already so pressed for time?"

Approached with a different attitude, the same issue is more likely to elicit a useful strategy. For example: "How can I rearrange my schedule to allow time for exercise (that will ultimately give me more energy to work more effectively)?"

For every obstacle you can identify, try a re-frame. See it as a challenge to find a way of overcoming it. Write down a few. At times certain things might work better than others. An obstacle to losing weight might be the long business lunches that are part of your job. Several strategies might suggest themselves – arrange the meeting in some other social setting (a game of golf might sound clichéd but it avoids high kilojoule consumption), or choose a restaurant that you know will serve a low-fat option.

The smaller obstacles are the daily events that can crop up and play havoc with your good intentions. These are easier to deal with and the strategy could include a contingency plan. For example, if a meeting goes overtime on Wednesday and you can't get to the gym, walk for 40 minutes on Thursday morning instead.

- What will get in the way?
- What are some ways of overcoming this?

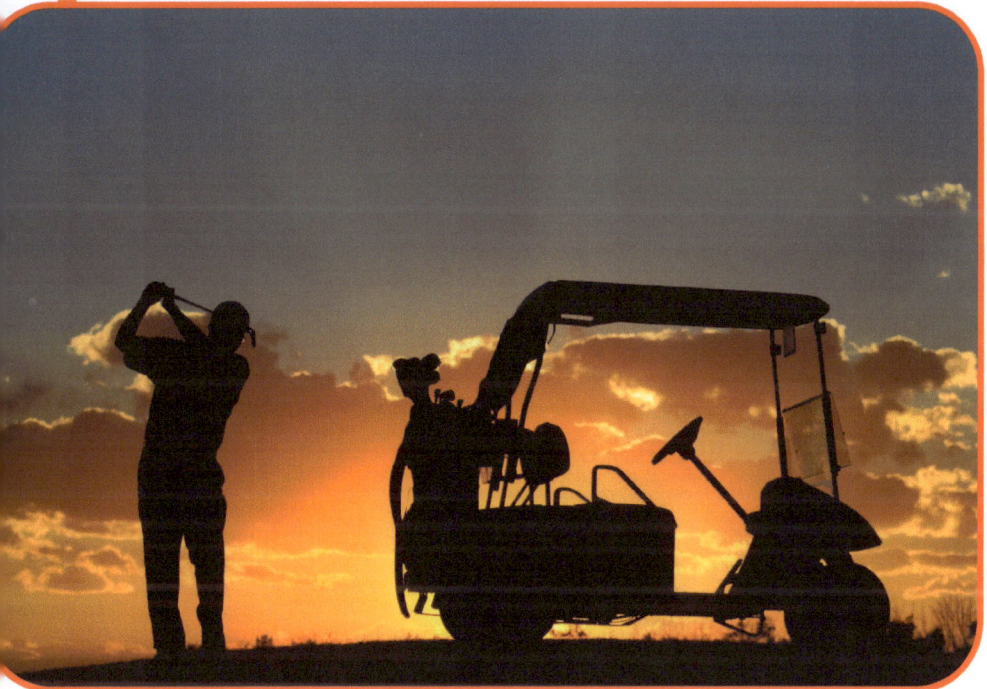

These first five building blocks create the base of the pyramid – its foundations. Without them, the plan is in danger of failing. This first layer helps you create the vision we touched on earlier.

With a wellness vision in place the next stage is to prepare fully for action. More planning is required at this stage and this can be broken into more building blocks, each one just as important as the next.

PREPARATION

Goals and plan

So you know what you want to achieve. How are you going to get there? This is where a detailed description of the action you plan to take is essential. You can break down your behaviour change into small, manageable steps. What do you want to be doing by when? Look at a three-month plan and weekly goals. We will cover goal setting in more detail in coming chapters. For now, you need a plan because without one, you will not make your vision a reality.

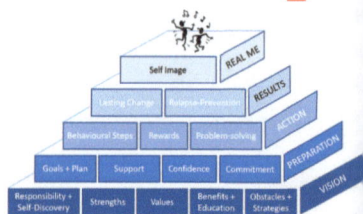

"What will I be doing in three months time that will be different?"

"What can I do each week to work towards that slowly and steadily?"

Three-month goals:

- I will be running three times a week

- I will only have 2 glasses of wine four nights a week

- I will have joined weight watchers

Weekly goals:

- I will have 2 alcohol-free days this week
- I will meet with John and ask him about how he lost his weight
- I will walk Monday and Wednesday lunchtimes for 45 minutes

Support

How will you gain support for your plan? What do you need in the way of support? Enlisting the help of friends and family increases your chances of success. You may not need much from them. You may ask that they "stay off your back" and not continually check on how you're going. Every one of us is different in what we find supportive. So don't expect people to read your mind. Ask for what you need.

"I am planning to give up smoking. Can you not smoke in front of me please?"

"I am going to lose some weight. Can you avoid buying chocolate biscuits for the family?"

"I would like to get fitter. Would you be willing to walk with me regularly?"

Then there is another form of support; the kind you can get from outside agencies, programs or providers. Do you need to follow a stop-smoking program? Is there a weight-loss group you wish to join? Do you need a personal trainer or nutritionist? Would a stress test be a useful thing to have as a starting point? Do you want to join a local health club, sports group, running club or similar? Being able to work out how to get the help you need is a major step towards change.

Confidence

By doing everything you can to be as fully prepared as possible, you will increase your feelings of confidence about success. The work you have done already will show you that you do have the base upon which you can build a successful change plan.

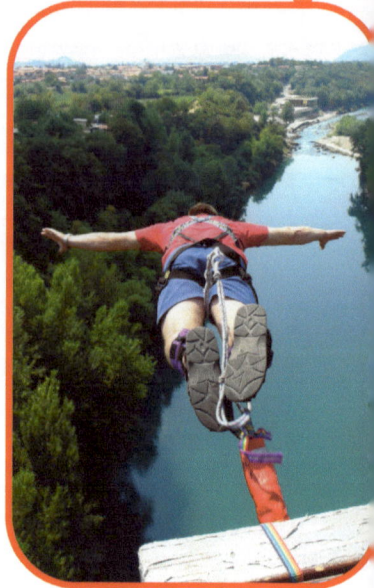

Of course, it can be difficult to sustain a feeling of total confidence about making major lifestyle changes. You may be holding on to past failures or doubts that need to be worked through, but the first step is to feel confident that you can achieve the initial goals you set for yourself. And this is where you begin. Choose an action that you know you can complete. If you can get your confidence to seven out of 10 then you are likely to succeed with that goal. If it is not that high yet, go back to the other building blocks and restrengthen your resolve. Or consider changing your initial goals. It may be that you are trying for a big result too soon. Make sure that you are only taking steps that are well within your capabilities. Small successes will add to your confidence.

"How confident do I feel that I can succeed at this?"

"What will it take to increase my confidence?"

Commitment

It's crunch time. Everything you have done so far has been groundwork. When you have decided what it is you want to achieve, write it down. Say it aloud to someone else. Make your vision concrete. Print it out, frame it, display it, circulate it to the office (or at least show your family). You may well inspire someone else to change. If you are not a person who likes to share your private life, make sure you have your plan somewhere that you can see it easily. If you do like to share, tell the world, and tell them why. When you get to the goal-setting stage, write your goals down each week and own them. Because each week you will be answering to yourself and you need to be very clear and precise about what you have committed to.

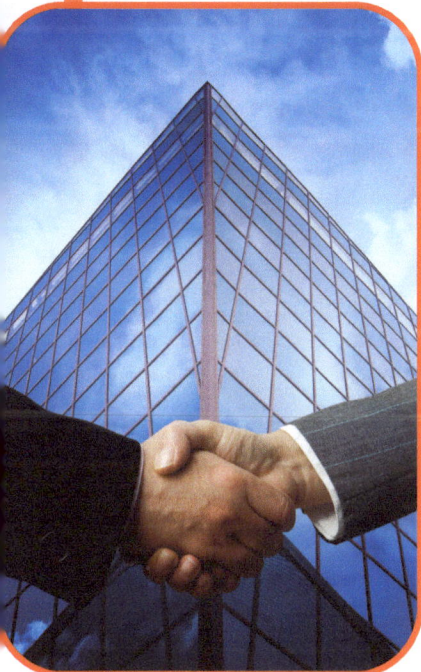

ACTION

Problem solving

Problem solving is the action you take in relation to obstacles. When you identified things that could prevent you from making the changes you want, you will also have thought of some strategies to use that will help you move forward. During this process you have actually begun to problem solve – a skill that you will use many times in the coming months. Becoming a successful problem solver will boost your confidence to overcome any future hurdles.

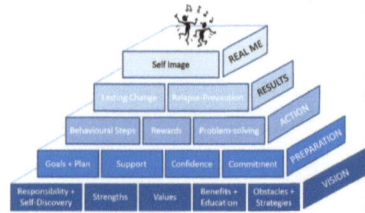

How can I look at this a different way?

What else could I do?

What are some other options?

Behavioural steps

Behavioural steps are the carefully designed actions you have decided to take to progress towards your vision. Your goals will consist of steps towards new behaviours that you wish to adopt that will result in the changes you desire. Commit to mastery of new behaviours in three months time and maintain them for a further three months. You will be well on your way to lasting change and to a new level of wellness.

Buy yourself a
bunch of flowers

Learn to self-talk
using praise and
congratulatory
terms

Have a massage

Recognise your
success!

Rewards

Rewards come in many shapes and sizes. You will learn quickly the satisfaction that comes from completing weekly goals. You will gain pleasure from the increased energy, reduced stress, better sleep patterns, weight loss, and feelings of vitality and control that you start to notice after a week or so. It is very important that you become mindful of these feelings and recognise them for what they are - evidence that you are making change and progress.

The ultimate reward will come when you are living well and making great choices most of the time. Along the way, you can learn to congratulate yourself on your achievements, however small.

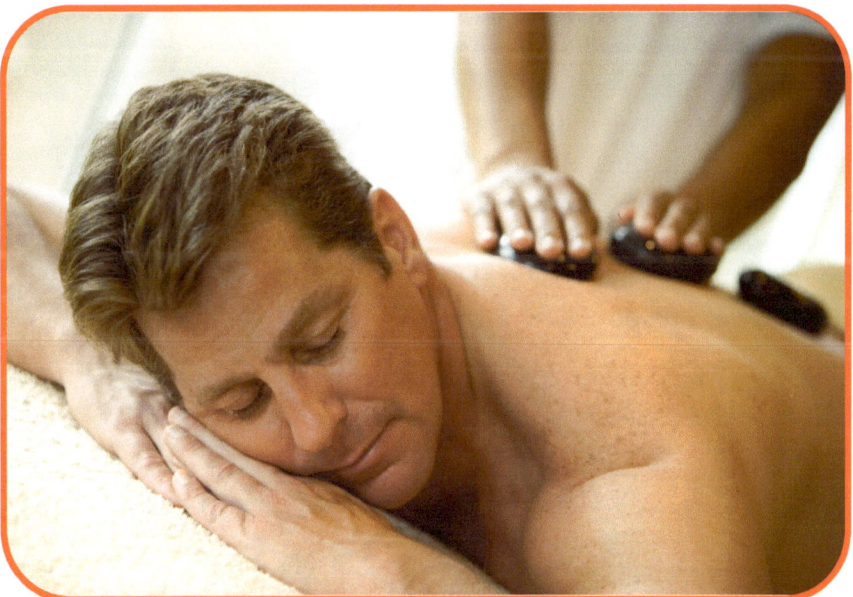

RESULTS

Lasting change

You are doing it! And you can keep living this way. What a great feeling. Enjoy the sense of achievement and mastery that comes with success. Only true effort and commitment can give you this, so congratulate yourself.

Relapse prevention

There will be situations that arise that are risky. Such circumstances have the potential to cause you to lose momentum or take a step backwards. By now you may well be in the maintenance stage of change, but forewarned is forearmed. It's a good idea to identify potential high risk circumstances and create a plan.

For example, if you have already thought about what you will eat at, say, Christmas dinner, this can give you the control you need to stay on track. You may decide that this one day a year could be a "let loose" day and that is a decision you have made in advance instead of being taken by surprise on the day and feeling that you have blown all your efforts. A very different response.

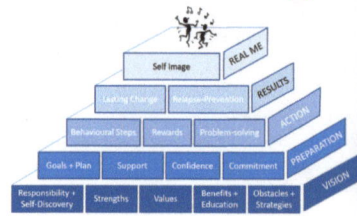

"I saw an angel in the stone and I carved to set her free."

Michelangelo

THE REAL ME

Best self

At the end of this journey, you will feel a strong sense of pride and achievement. Some changes are quite major and can create physical change as well as mental change, so it appears that you have found a new part of yourself, if not developed into a whole new person. Small changes can completely transform you because they flow on to so many other areas.

The NWCR found that people who managed to maintain their weight loss had undergone a "transformation", by finding a coach, mentor or guide, pulling back from their old environment and then being "reborn" into a different way of life. They became leaders rather than followers and frequently took on the role of helper in some capacity for someone else or a group in need.

Another finding was that they all engaged in some form of meditative activity that allowed them time to reflect and stand back from the old obsessive behaviour.

"The transformation of identity seems to be the crucial factor in keeping the weight off. The person finds a 'new self' and can then let go of their former tendency to engage in unhealthy habits."

Summary

- Change rarely progresses in a steady, linear direction. We often take two steps forward and one step back. Keep moving.

- Think of your change process as building a pyramid that's strong enough to climb and hold you steady at the top.

- The first step in making lasting change is to take responsibility for yourself.

- Understanding the role of values is important. Your deepest beliefs and principles inform your vision and motivate you to change.

- The preparation level requires confidence, commitment, planning and plenty of support. There is much thinking work to be done.

- During the action phase you will be doing a lot of problem solving as you overcome hurdles. It's important to reward yourself along the way.

- At the results level, make sure you have some relapse prevention strategies in place. Complacency is the enemy.

- At the pinnacle of the change pyramid is the real you, uncovered by a process of transformation.

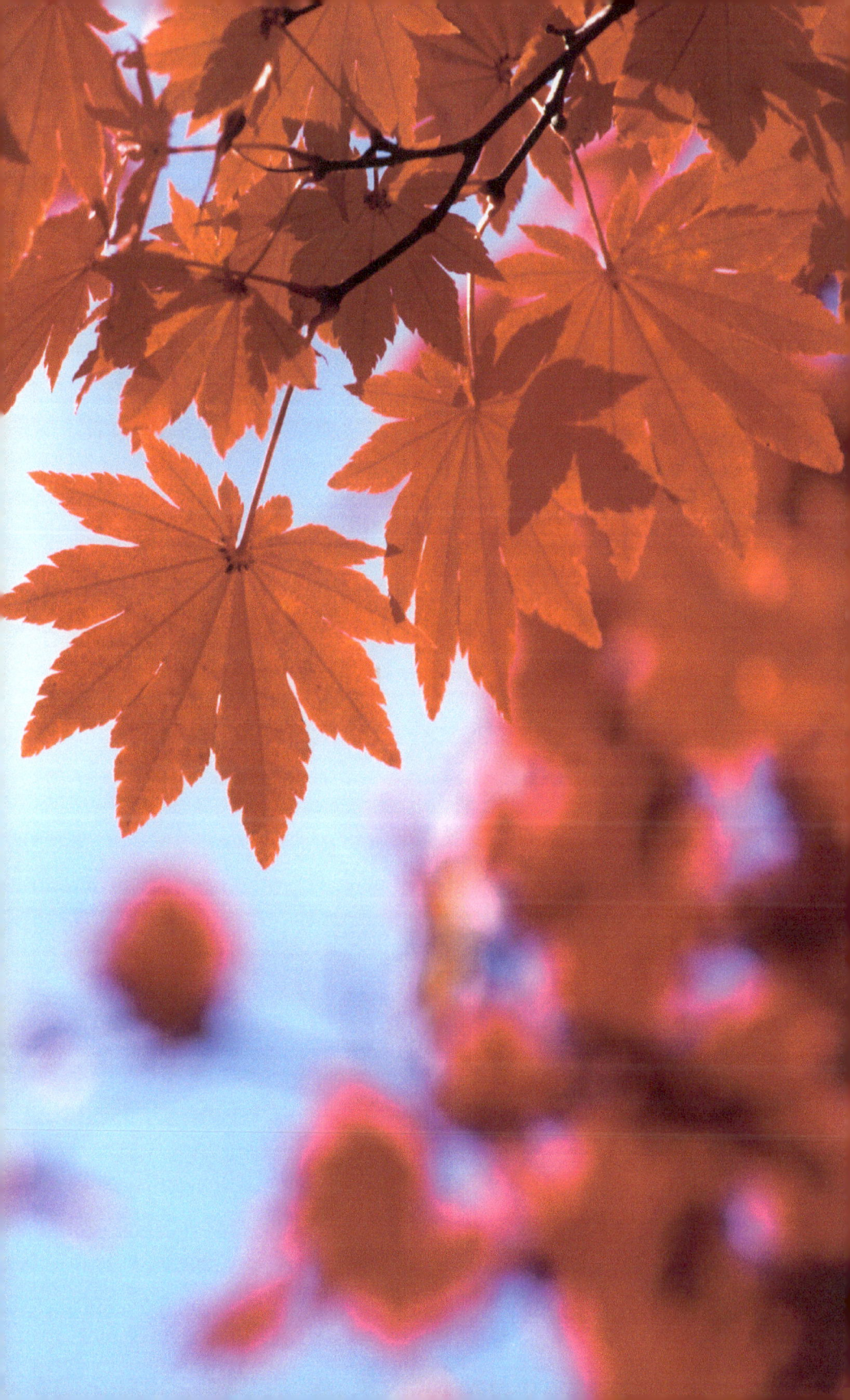

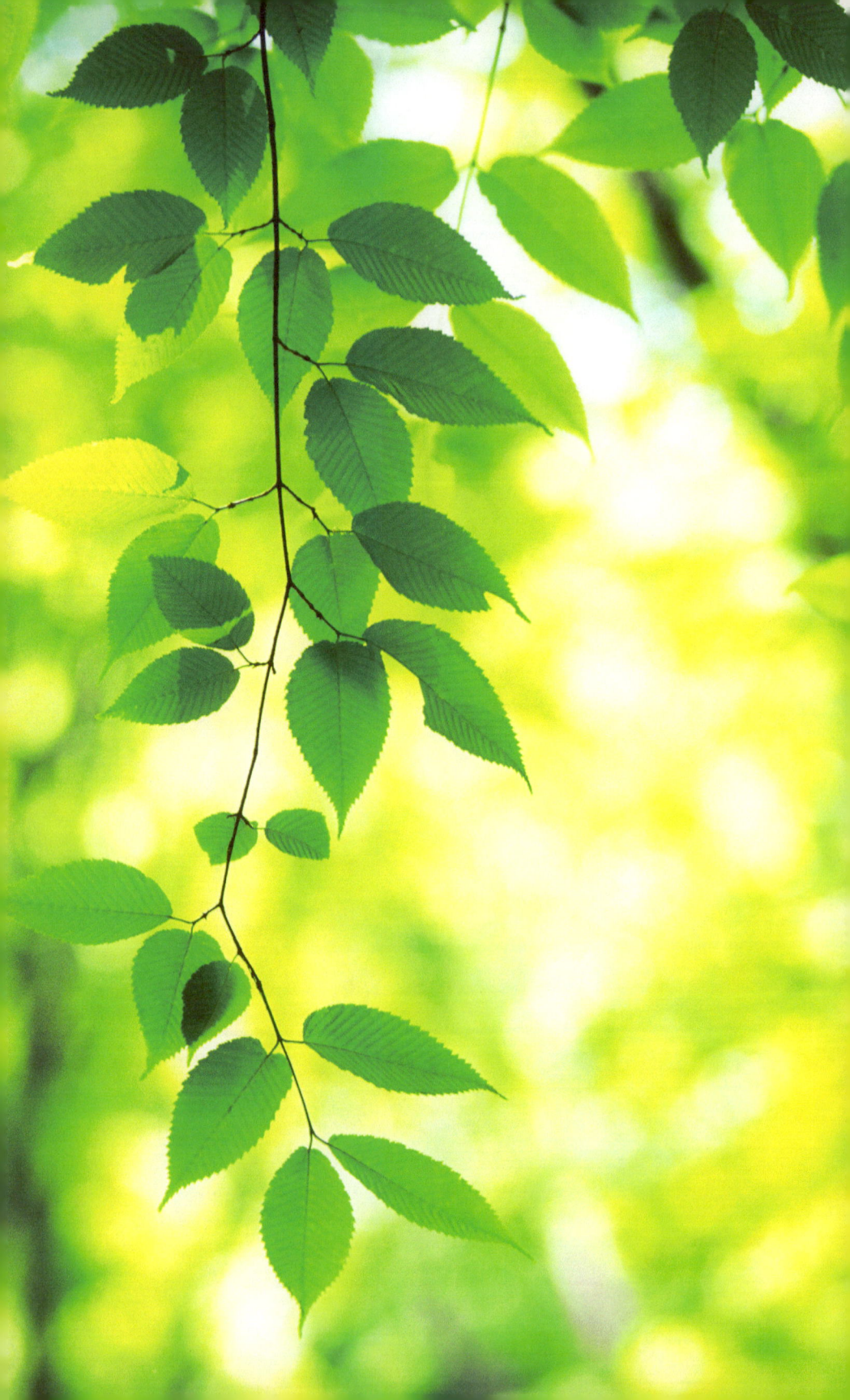

Section five

THE PLAN

How do you rate yourself as a person?

How you feel about yourself plays a very important role in the success of your plan to change towards greater wellness. For the purposes of this exercise, there are two parts to your self-assessment. Firstly, how you feel about yourself globally, that is your worth as a person, or self-esteem. Secondly, how capable you think you are of succeeding at this one given project: self-efficacy. Self-esteem and self-efficacy are connected in some ways though not necessarily in the way you might assume.

For example, if you think highly of yourself as a person, it does not mean that you feel you are any more capable of, say, jumping out of a plane, or standing up and giving a speech to year 12 school leavers. You might feel more confident in general than people who have low opinions of themselves, but the skills that are needed for the two tasks are quite separate and distinct from having a positive opinion of oneself as a person.

However, general confidence in yourself as a person and skill-based confidence are both important to success in making positive and lasting change. This is how they work.

In our earlier discussion about creating a wellness vision we noted the importance of taking an inventory of your strengths. This is a great place to start. Not only will this exercise help your self-esteem, it will also help your self-efficacy. Such a list can strengthen your belief that you do have what it takes to succeed in this change process, because the list represents the evidence.

By concentrating on what we have going for us, we create positive energy that sets the right climate for success. So take some time to review what you have achieved, what you are good at and what it took. The next step is to ask people around you what they consider are your unique strengths. Add them to the list. You may be surprised at what they come up with.

I believe I am:

Organised
Committed
Philosophical
Humorous
Fun to be with
Sensitive to other people
Determined
Thorough

Other people say I am:

A good friend
A perfectionist
A high achiever
Loyal

These may not seem to be totally relevant to your goals but you might be surprised at how these qualities can help in various ways. Take time out to consider how they may be of use. For example, "Fun to be with" could translate to "I should be able to find an exercise buddy easily".

If you need some expert prompting with this, try the Web. The University of Pennsylvania's Positive Psychology Centre offers an online survey which identifies character strengths. You can find its VIA Inventory of Strengths Survey at http://www.viasurvey.org/.

Set aside a week for keeping a journal of success and wins. At the end of each day in that week, write down what you did well or what went well during that day. There is always something. If you find this esteeming, why stop after a week?

Come up with a comprehensive description of yourself that states quite clearly where your strengths lie and put it somewhere you can see easily. Keep adding to it. This is a great exercise to do in the preparation phase so that you start with a feeling of confidence and are armed with a clear picture of who you are and what those unhealthy habits are up against.

Research suggests that if we can look positively at the past, present and future, our self-esteem will grown.

Feeling grateful for all the good experiences

Today, I:

Slept in… and felt better rested!

Finished the report I was working on

Enjoyed 10 minutes in the sun at lunchtime

"Gratitude is the ability to appreciate again and again, freshly, naively, the basic goods of life with awe, pleasure and wonder."

Abraham Maslow

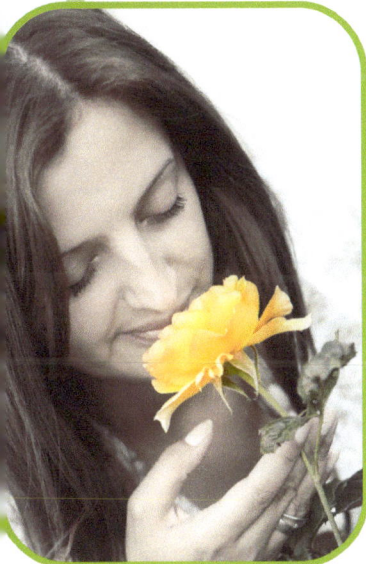

we have had can shift our thinking quite dramatically. Try making another list.

Learning to forgive people for the hurt they have caused us can relieve weight from our shoulders we didn't even know we were carrying. Writing a letter that you may or may not send can be a very healing process – even if the person you are writing to is no longer around, write a letter anyway. Forgiving does not make their actions right, it just takes the burden of resentment away.

The present is really what life is all about. Learning to appreciate the moment and becoming more aware of what is happening around us, how we are feeling and what pleasure, if any, is being experienced, can change our attitude to life remarkably. Slow down to start.

The future holds promise of exciting things to come. Anticipation and planning can create enormous pleasure, which is why we start with a vision for our ideal health. Start enjoying the feeling of what it could be like now. The flip side to this is unnecessary worry. This can take more work but when you read the section on negative thinking you will be better equipped to handle your own "gremlins".

As your self-esteem increases, so will your ability to bounce back after setbacks.

Increasing your belief that you can succeed

Self-efficacy is a fascinating concept. If we do not believe we are capable of completing a task, chances are we will be anxious and less inclined to put in the effort required. Fortunately, there are tactics for increasing our self-efficacy that can really help.

Congratulate yourself

When you are acting as your own coach, you need to learn how to encourage yourself and promote your own confidence. The simplest way to do this is to set yourself a task that is achievable. It may take some effort but does not stretch you in a way that might produce failure. Once you have completed this task, take time out to pat yourself on the back and say "Well done".

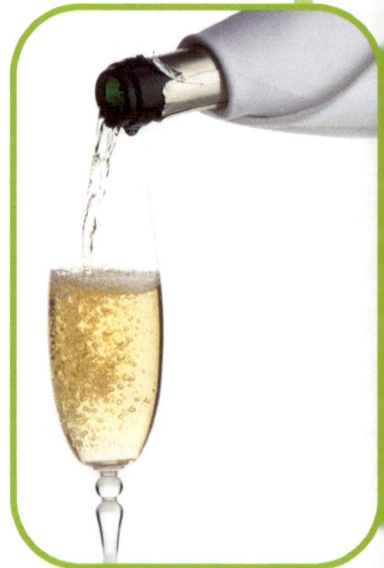

Some years ago, I had to give a talk to a fairly challenging audience of men in a profession that was not known for its humour or broadmindedness. The subject of the talk was "How to get and maintain a positive attitude". My style was to use humour and warmth to create laughter and, hopefully, learning. I was surprised by how well the talk went and when I left the room following loud applause, I felt a burst of pride and satisfaction, closely followed by the realisation that there was not one person in the room who I knew or would likely see again. Nor did I have a partner at that time who was waiting for my phone call to tell him how it went. So who knew I did a good job? That day I learnt to congratulate myself and spent 30 minutes before returning to work, rewarding myself by reliving the experience and basking in the memory of the audience's response.

Physiological states

If our bodies reflect our emotions, is it possible to change what's happening in our bodies, and then let our feelings follow? Put another way, if we are stressed and our muscles are tense, will relaxing them help us feel calmer? The answer is, of course.

Learning to get in touch with what your physiological state is, and making changes if necessary, can be very helpful in increasing self-efficacy. This has worked with athletes and performers for years, why not everyone else? Have you ever felt really down and depressed and noticed how you are sitting or what your posture represents? Next time you become aware of that, try this. Stand up straight, put your shoulders back, your chin up, adopt a determined air and say loudly, "I AM SO DEPRESSED!" It's hard to stay down when you're smiling.

Learning to control your body can have an incredibly liberating impact on your mood. This is why exercise can be so very useful in preventing depression.

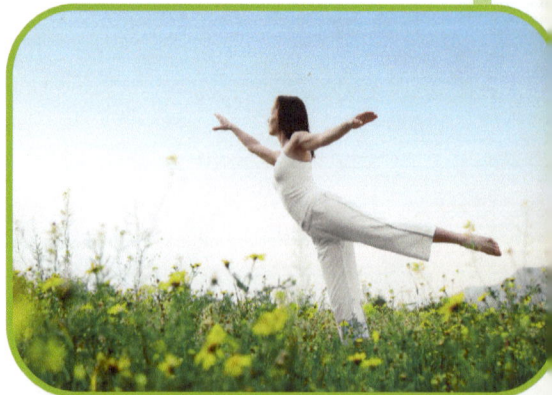

eople with a high level
f personal mastery live
n a continual learning
mode. They never
'arrive'. Sometimes,
anguage, such as the
rm 'personal mastery',
creates a misleading
nse of definiteness, of
black and white.

But personal mastery
s not something you
ossess. It is a process.
is a lifelong discipline.
eople with a high level
of personal mastery
are acutely aware of
their ignorance, their
incompetence, their
growth areas.

Paradoxical? Only for
hose who do not see
hat the journey is the
reward."

eter Senge, in The 5th
Discipline

Vicarious experiences – watching others

There is nothing more powerful for increasing your belief that something can be done, than seeing someone else doing it. Makeover shows, success stories and testimonials all demand attention and have a very positive effect on the reader or viewer. "If they can do it, then so can I." The closer the person is to you and the more you respect them, the greater the impact their success will have on you. Surround yourself with those people - or at least spend time with them.

Mastery experiences

I lied. There is one thing that is more powerful – your own successes. We return to the need to take small, achievable steps so we can experience the clocking up of successes. Again, revisit your past achievements and bask in the glow of remembered accomplishment.

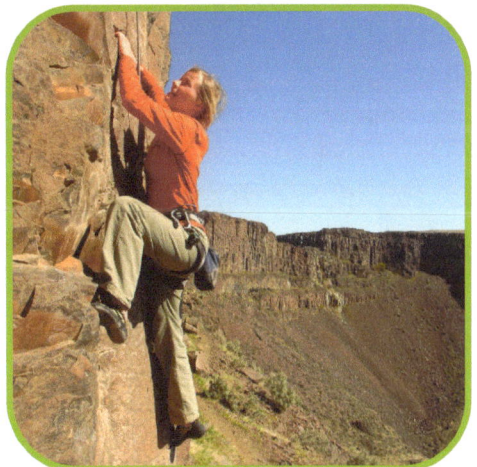

Creating a plan to achieve your goals

Now you have worked through many different aspects of what you would like to change in your wellness, it is time to make a plan. You have the vision, you know why it is important to you, you know what could get in the way and you've come up with some strategies for overcoming those obstacles.

You know why change is difficult and you appreciate the value of taking small easy steps. So the next question is:

What specific behaviours would you like to be doing consistently in three months time that will be moving you actively in the direction of your vision?

These behaviours constitute the action plan. They are actions and ways of being that are consistent with your new lifestyle. They are the new wellness habits you want to develop.

You may wonder why three months is the chosen time frame. Why not six months, one month, a year? The answer is simple. It is important to have enough time to work towards those new behaviours, step by step; and it is also important to create a certain sense of urgency for action and for weekly goal setting. Three months strikes a good balance between the two.

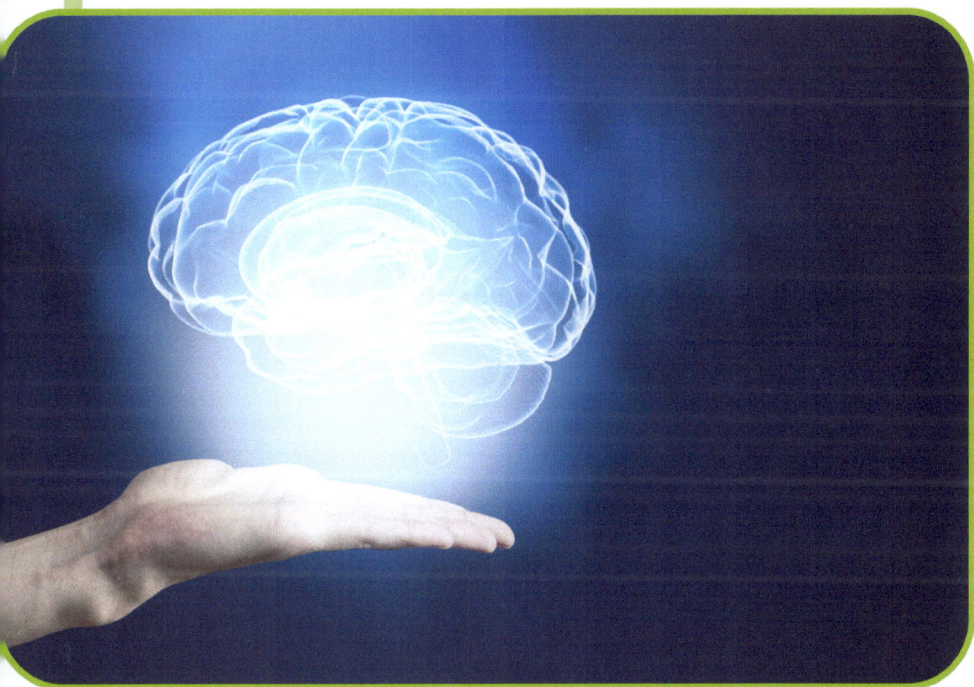

Why are goals necessary?

Goals represent milestones on a journey. If you don't have small, achievable, concrete steps to take, there is no pathway forward. While motivation and self-esteem provide the push, goals provide the pull.

Goal setting is an area that has attracted a great deal of research. Which goals are best? What degree of difficulty should they have? How many should you set? This will be answered shortly, but the most important thing about goals is that they make you plan.

Ever heard of SMART goals? For a goal to be effective, it must fit into the following criteria:

S – specific. If a goal is too vague, how do you know if you have reached it? For example, "I will be more active this week", or, "I will be training regularly in three months time"? More active than what? What does training mean?

M – measurable. To be effective, a goal must have something about it that can be measured. Training regularly might mean three times a week or five times a week, and for how long at what intensity? Ideally, you should state what days of the week, how long each training session will last and what intensity and activity will be performed. Goal setting allows us to measure success and progress.

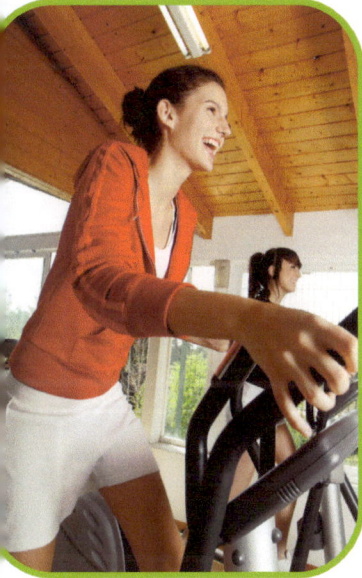

A – action oriented. The goal must also have action built into it. Even if it is a "thinking" goal it needs to be tied to an action. So instead of "I will think about why I want to reduce my working hours", make the goal, "I will list reasons for wanting to reduce my working hours". Just remember the golden rule of goals – they need to describe actions or behaviours.

R – realistic. A difficult goal can be good; we call them "stretch" goals. They're the ones that make you work a bit harder and give a greater sense of achievement. However, since a policy of small, easy steps is integral to the success of this program, achieving the goals you set yourself needs to actually be possible. A goal of running seven days of the week, for example, is not realistic. Something would break down, and quickly, if this is a new activity and the only experience is failure.

T – time framed. Weekly goals, three monthly goals, daily goals are examples of time framing your plan. Walking for 45 minutes on Monday, Wednesday and Friday is another.

The goal needs to **be tied into whatever outcome** you desire. So when you're going on your walks, for example, you know that this will result in more energy, more kilojoule output and enhanced relaxation. If those are elements of your vision, then the goal makes sense. If they are not, then why do it?

Designing three-month goals

These goals are sets of behaviours that you wish to be doing in three months time. They will move you towards your vision but they are not the vision itself.

So if your vision is to have more vitality by being fitter and stronger so that you can fully engage in your children's activities, your three-month goals will consist of behaviours that will get you fitter and stronger.

A good three-month goal might be:

I will be following a 20-minute strength-training routine covering all major muscle groups of my body on three days of the week.

A poor three-month goal would say:

I will be stronger from going to the gym.

Get it?

Step one is to define the elements of your vision.

For example:

- Weight control
- Healthy eating
- Fitness

Then, under each of those headings, define sets of behaviours that will achieve what you want.

Weight control –

- I will lose 3kg by following the exercise and nutrition plan below.

Healthy eating –

- I will substitute a piece of fresh fruit for dessert five days of the week, allowing myself dessert on the weekends only.

- I will drink no more than two glasses of wine on four days of the week with no alcohol on the remaining three days.

- I will take my lunch to work three days of the week, making a healthy low-fat sandwich or salad the night before.

Fitness –

- I will become a member of my local gym and attend three times a week to do one cycling class, one pump class and one circuit class.

- I will be using a personal trainer to help me with a strength routine twice a week.

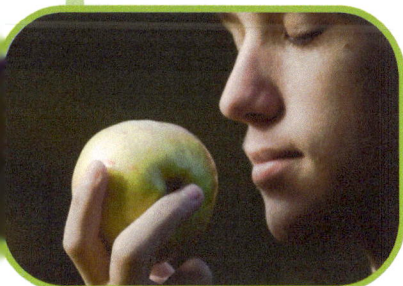

Examples of how the above goals could be written poorly:

Weight control

- I will lose 10kg.

Unrealistic in three months and no action tied to it. How?

Healthy eating

- *I will cut down on kilojoules*

How many? How can we measure this?

Fitness

- *I will be running regularly and be fitter than I am now.*

How fast, how often? How will you know you are fitter than you are now?

It is quite easy to set poorly defined goals. Take time with the wording and ask yourself about each goal:

- What will this achieve?
- Will it give me the desired result?
- Is it something that I want to do?
- Are the rewards bigger than the effort?
- Are my chances of success more than 70%?

Setting weekly goals

This is truly the beginning. By now you have thought through your plan and will be clearer about the steps that need to be taken and how you can start work on building your pyramid with a strong foundation. Your first weekly goals may be related to gaining support, finding more information about risks and benefits, and working out the logistics regarding what is possible and achievable for you with your current lifestyle. Your commitment to your plan will be high. So set yourself up for success.

You may decide that some elements of your vision require two or three goals. Go through the same process we used for defining the three-monthly goals.

Let's take the same example:

Weight control

No goal needed. The aim is to slowly start the behaviours that will result in weight loss. Weekly weighing is not the way to go.

Healthy eating

- *I will eat a piece of fresh fruit for dessert on Monday.*

  Comment: I will warn the kids they will have to get their own dessert.

- *I will go for a walk at 6pm on Wednesday when I get home from work.*

Comment: This will replace my habit of having a glass of wine.

Fitness

- *I will find out membership prices at the gym by going in on Thursday night on my way home from work.*
- *I will call Tanya to see if she can take any ore personal training clients.*
- *I will walk for 30 minutes in the park before work on Tuesday and Thursday morning.*

And ask the same questions:

- What will this achieve?
- Will it give me the desired result?
- Is it something that I want to do?
- Are the rewards bigger than the effort?
- Are my chances of success more than 70%?

If the answers aren't positive, change the goal.

The next questions to ask are:

- What could get in the way?
- What are some strategies to deal with this possibility?
- How committed am I to do this?

Go through this process each week as you set new goals.

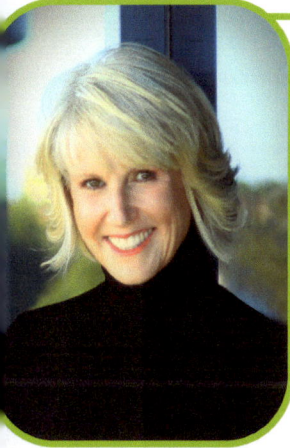

My journey to wellness cannot be told without touching on recent life events.

There is no second chance at dying, but living is a different matter. I was diagnosed with a critical illness and experienced an allergic reaction to chemotherapy which was daunting to say the least. I know many people would have expected me to react in fear. However, my faith allowed me to realise that I do not fear death, rather I fear not being able to live fully. I believe it is this zest for life and determination to not disappear inside the pain of what was happening to me that allowed me to remain focused to return myself, with the help of my medical team, back to perfect wellness which has now taken on a whole new significance.

During my treatment I had no control over anything other than the way I chose to experience life. I think prior to this time I would have completed my morning rituals of meditation and exercise before embarking on a super busy time filling my days with some stuff that to be honest is not totally important. Now I watch the sunrise without trying to capture it on the phone - I want to experience it. I'm living in a way that supports my health - in mind, body and soul. I love journaling my insights after meditation and appreciate the small things that make life special - beautiful conversations, sunshine, being in nature and the wonderful opportunity to work creatively. It is being fully conscious within the present moment that I believe allows us to step away from fear and into courage to allow us to navigate through any situation.

This chapter of my life has allowed me to recognise in a powerful way that we are all individuals, not statistics that are walking the same path. My lesson was to enjoy every moment for the joy of its experience or the value of what it taught me.

I believe the timing of life is perfect and always has been. Let each day forward unfold as it should. I will be forever grateful for what I have learnt through my journey with cancer as it has allowed me to experience true wellness.

Fellow & Accredited Interior Designer of The Design Institute of Australia, Founder & Creative Director of The Interior Space, Author & Speaker.

Website – www.theinteriorspace.com.au; Email – ros@theinteriorspace.com.au
Ros Hemley, FDIA, CKD Au, MCES

Creating a structure of accountability

So you're on the way. The fun begins, and so do the challenges.

When you feel confident that you have created well thought-out and worded goals, it's time to think ahead to your weekly self-coaching session. If you can set a regular time to do this, it does make it easier. Block it out in your diary and take 15 minutes to review the week. Your self-interview might go something like this:

How has my week been? What successes and wins did I have?

How is my mood right now? Am I feeling positive or negative? How is my energy? If low, what could I do to change that? (Maybe take five minutes to unwind and focus).

Now it's time for goal review.

Go through each goal and ask:

- Did I achieve that goal?
- What went well? What not so well?
- What did it feel like when it went well?
- Was there anything I could have done differently when that obstacle came up?
- What did I learn?
- What percentage of that goal did I achieve?

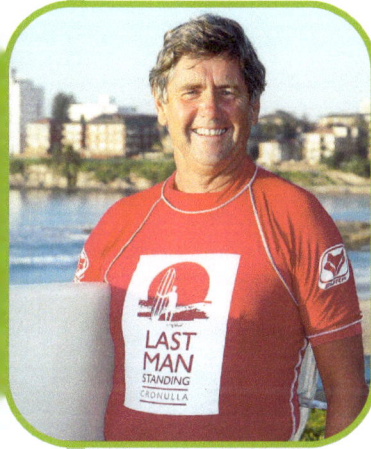

When you have gone through each goal carefully, now ask:

What would I like to do next?

- Are these goals still working for me?
- Do I want to set new goals?
- Are they still keeping me on track for my three-monthly goals?
- Is there anything else I can do to keep my commitment high and increase my chances of success?
- Is the satisfaction of achieving what I set out to do enough, or can I reward myself for my efforts in another way?

"Many years ago I decided to make exercise part of my day, not in addition to my day. That is why I start the morning at the beach … for a run, walk or surf. I enjoy the buddy system of participation rather than the loner approach. Why do I do what I do?

- I am conscious of the standard I set as a leader at work.
- To outlive my parents who died too young (57 & 63).
- To watch my kids grow up & be part of their life.
- To provide my kids with a fun environment to live in that is not available to everyone, and was not available to my wife and myself."

Terry Dewing, a business developer who has completed 27 Sutherland to Surf community runs of 11km. Terry surfs, runs, rides and skis

Bouncing back after setbacks – the importance of resilience

- **How you think about your successes and failures**

If you enjoy success and tell yourself you were "lucky", you don't really take the credit for your achievement. Similarly, if you make a mistake or fail to reach a goal and tell yourself something like "I never get it right", you are taking the opposing extreme view of too much responsibility. Can you see how this can work against self-esteem? Become aware of what you are telling yourself each time you either achieve, or fail to achieve. Try to adjust your responsibility meter to take credit where it's due and to recognise appropriately, not catastrophically, when you did perhaps go wrong. Do not put the blame completely on outside influences and do not give away the opportunity to congratulate yourself when it is your due.

If you have a week when you fail to meet a goal you have set, remember that the behaviour you chose suited you at the time (which is why we do anything). It may have been an old pattern, it may have been an overwhelming desire to eat that dessert, to stay in bed or stay out too late. That was your choice in that moment. We have no influence on the past but we can choose to take action in the present and plan for the future. So cut your losses, fairly evaluate what you did or did not do that week, and either revise your goals for next week or plan to change the circumstances that prompted the incompatible behaviour.

- **Replace negative with positive thoughts**

When you catch yourself in your negative thoughts like, "I knew I couldn't do it", internally shout "Stop!" Replace the negative statement with something more realistic, such as "I knew it wasn't going to be easy but I am strong and determined to succeed."

Keep doing this every time you find yourself in self-berating mode.

- **The ability to review and learn**

We all make mistakes. Allow yourself a few in life and view them as learning opportunities.

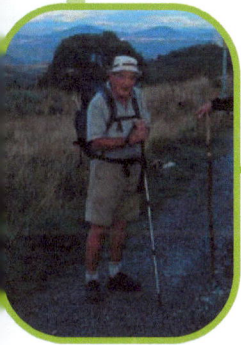

"I wanted to see Spain so decided that the best way to do that was to walk it. My motivation to keep fit and active? Simple – I don't want to die in bed. I have certain physical limitations but I will not let them destroy my life. I can't choose how I die but I can choose how I live."

Stan at 76. He walked 751km from Roncevelles to Santiago in 2006 over five weeks and over some of the most mountainous terrain in Europe. Stan has suffered from emphysema, aortic fibrillation, severe foot problems and epilepsy. He trained at the gym and when he began training his heart was 50% enlarged. He reduced it to normal size. Stan's motto was, "To thine own self be true."

Summary

- Self-esteem and self-efficacy are equally important in creating the positive energy we need to sustain change.

- You can increase your belief in your capacity to succeed by congratulating yourself for achieving small, do-able tasks and being conscious of what's going on with your body.

- The success of others can be very inspiring; even more powerful are memories of our own past successes.

- To bring your vision to life you need an action plan and concrete, measurable goals.

- Set weekly self-coaching sessions with yourself and review progress on your goals. It's all part of your accountability structure.

- Develop resilience by taking a measured view of progress and setbacks. Beating yourself up will only serve to undermine your self-esteem.

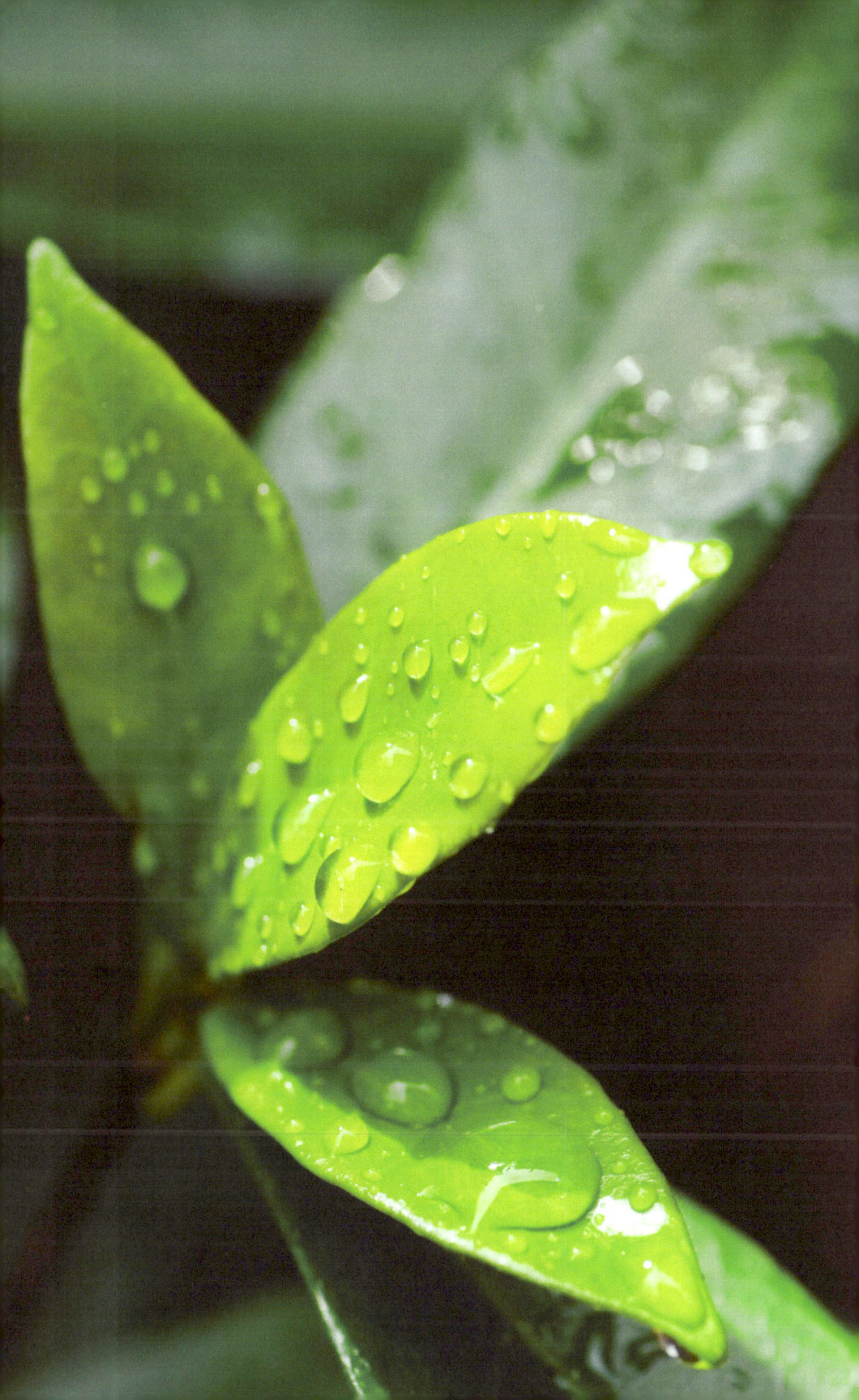

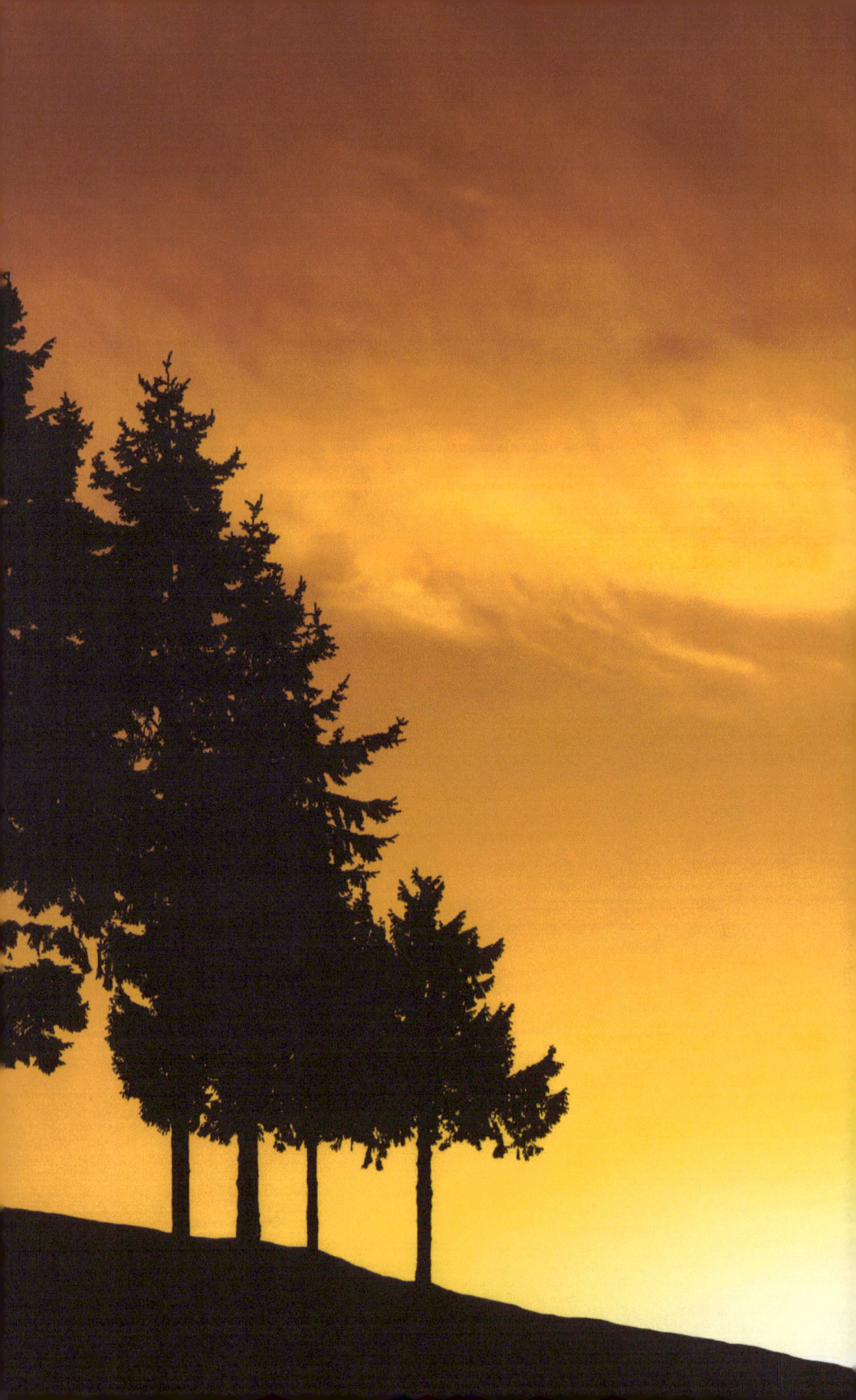

Section six

THE KEY TO SUCCESS

Building your support team

It is always easier to do anything in life when you have a good team on your side.

As we learnt in the pyramid model, support is among the essential building blocks. It will be different for everyone. Some people need more encouragement from outside. Others require detailed information. Some prefer to go it alone and have minimal reliance on others.

The following lists ideas that have been helpful to people going through lifestyle change. Pick those that appeal to you.

Family and friends

Do you need to tell them? Would you like to invite anyone to join you in your efforts? An exercise buddy can be very useful in getting you out of bed as you have the commitment to meet them.

Health club

Over the years, I have seen how valuable a good club can be for so many people. It satisfies one of the most basic of human needs – the need for belonging or affiliation. It also can give us the opportunity to take part in group activities, provide a structure for our exercise routine and put us in touch with a network of helping professionals. Personal trainers, nutritionists, massage therapists and even just familiar faces at the front desk can all play a part in our success.

Personal trainer

You can be trained in a club or outside, or in your house if you prefer. Finding the right match for your personality is essential. Choose carefully and your trainer can get you through the tough times.

Other groups and professional services

Consider the following:

- Weight Loss programs
- Quit smoking programs
- Running groups
- Bush walking clubs
- Cycling clubs
- Yoga and Pilates classes
- Personal Organisers

Dietitians, Nutritionists, Physiotherapists, Exercise Physiologists, Psychologists, Naturopaths, Osteopaths and Chiropractors are only a few of the supporting professional services you can use. All of these services exist for a reason. They work.

Groups can provide social support, safety, experience, knowledge, commitment and motivation. Research thoroughly, choose carefully. They could change your life.

Keeping your vision in sight

You are now on the path to a new stage of health and wellness. Perhaps you've read this book cover to cover - or you just delved in here and there to see what is involved. Whichever way you have approached it, you will be somewhere in the stages of change cycle; possibly at different stages for different health patterns.

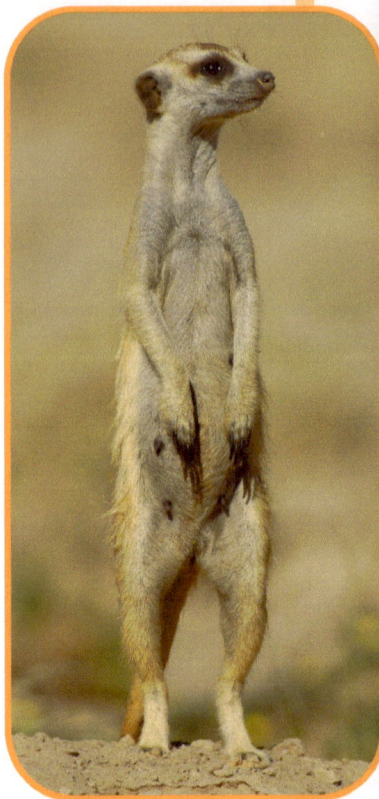

Keep Your Vision In Sight

Write it out, illustrate it if you can, keep returning to it, feel the way it can grab you with excitement and feed your determination. And never give up!

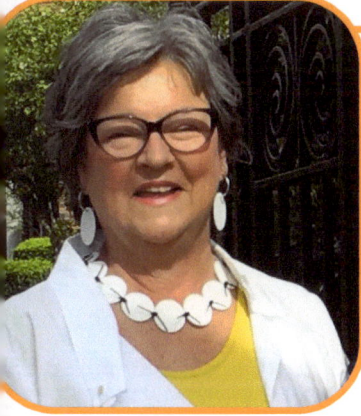

Chronic Fatigue Syndrome & Fibromyalgia brought my independent, active and social life to a complete standstill. It was a confronting diagnosis but, because I had felt so unwell for so long, it was a relief to know what I needed to battle. I was unable to work and rarely had enough energy to leave my house. I would save my strength to see my wonderfully supportive family, a few very close friends and my doctor. Certainly not how I would choose to live and I wanted to change this as soon as I possibly could.

It is always said that good health is the single most important part of life but very few of us really understand this until we are faced with a serious health scare.

Despite what I had read about this condition, I was determined, with every fibre of my being, that I would reclaim my life. If I couldn't eradicate this health problem, then I would manage it as best I could and enjoy my life to the full…maybe not everyone's full…but to my 'new' full.

I started with exercise, literally one step at a time…at first only a few metres… then a week or so later…a few more metres. Gradually I was able to build this up and, after a almost a year, I added aquarobics. I'm still doing aquarobics because I find the water very therapeutic. I've also added walking and regular visits to a small, friendly gym.

In conjunction with exercise, I changed my diet and prepared simpler, cleaner and healthier food; generally fresh, seasonal fruit & vegetables with a small amount of protein. These meals tasted better and I knew exactly what I was eating and how my meals were prepared. I was happy to accept this as my responsibility. I kept reminding myself of why I was making these changes and this kept me on track. I wanted my life to be as good as I could make it!

Ten years later, I've retired from full time work but I continue to lead a busy life and manage my Chronic Fatigue now by early awareness of a few important triggers, mainly balancing my energy levels rather than any specific maintenance. I also support this by continuing my healthy eating and exercise regimes, not always perfectly, but within tolerances I've come to understand work for my body.

In so doing, I have achieved a very happy lifestyle that allows me to add more exciting adventures and activity, so I am now able to deal confidently with anything the universe, or my friends, throw at me!

Robbie Durst
January 2018

Summary

Here is a quick overview of the material we've covered to get you on your way.

Write your vision

- **Who would you be at your best?**

- **What does it involve that is different?**

- **Why is that important to you?**

- **Make it full and cover all elements of your health**

- **Dig deep to uncover why you want those things**

Be honest about the obstacles that could get in the way

- **List them all**

Come up with strategies for overcoming the obstacles

Work out which stage of change you are at

Look at the things that can help move you forward

- **Write a Decisional Balance Sheet**

- **Get more information**

- **Refer to Mount Lasting Change and colour in the blocks as you work on each one**

What will you be doing that is different in three months time that will be moving you towards your vision?

- Remember this is time to identify specific behaviours for all elements of your vision

- It does not have to be the final picture but a big enough change to get you excited

What can you do immediately?

- Detailed planning begins

- What are your first week's goals?

- Three month goals and weekly goals need to be SMART

- Be ruthless in re-writing goals until they are precise, action oriented, you feel confident in meeting them and they get you where you want to be

Spend some time thinking about how you feel about yourself and your ability to succeed

- Is there any work you can do to increase your positive feelings about yourself?

- Can you begin to stop the negative self talk?

- List your past successes and your strengths

- Learn to congratulate yourself and forgive yourself when things don't go perfectly

A word on energy

A book on wellness would not be complete without a mention of energy.

Increased energy is often one of the advantages that people enjoy when they make changes in their lifestyles and it is certainly possible to achieve. By increasing fitness, decreasing stress and eating nutritious foods, your physical energy will be optimised. However, over the years I have seen many people whose physical energy is great but their other energy sources are depleted.

What are these other energy sources? Let's take a look:

- Physical energy
- Emotional energy
- Mental energy
- Spiritual energy

If we break these down further to determine where they all come from, it becomes easy to understand how they play a part in our overall energy status.

Physical energy relates to physiological states of fitness: how much oxygen we can carry to the working muscles, how quickly we recover from exertion, how strong each muscle group is and how much fuel is available to produce this energy. The more active we are the higher our physical energy is, as long as there is no other physical condition which might affect our functioning.

Emotional energy is determined by how positive we are feeling at any given time. Family and friends are often influential. In fact relationships of any kind play a part, including work relationships. Striking a balance between work and play is important. Laughter, appreciation, gratitude, love and empathy will all increase emotional energy.

Mental energy is directly proportional to how much you are being challenged or stimulated. Do you find your work rewarding and have opportunities for new tasks and ideas? Are you involved in decision-making? Is there an atmosphere in your workplace that is conducive to change or are people threatened by it?

Spiritual energy is the most important. If you think about what you value in life and then ask yourself if you are living in a way that is in tune with those values, then it's likely your spiritual energy will be high. If, however, you are not, then you will be having some internal conflict which may present itself in different ways but will always lead to a sense of discontent. So, if loyalty is high on your list of values and you are cheating on your partner, chances are you will be low on spiritual energy. If you value fun and laughter and your workplace is full of serious people who do not share any humour, then your working day will be low in this energy source.

Look carefully at your workplace

We spend a lot of time at work. I have often seen people content in their personal life but "putting up" with work. Often the reasons seem to fit in one of the categories we have looked at above. If you value physical fitness and your workplace has no health promotion policy, then it's not a good fit. If the feeling at work is that top management do not really care about their employees and there is little team atmosphere, then emotional energy will be at a low. If the company does not have a mission statement, or there is no clear idea of what the company stands for, then spiritual energy suffers. If people resist change and there is a culture of letting things slide, then mental energy is likely to be minimal.

And in your personal life

Next take a good look at your life outside of work. Make sure that you are using all four energy sources and that there isn't one area that needs attention. Unless you are drawing on all four sources, it is unlikely you will enjoy a sense of being fully engaged in your life.

Personal organisation

This has become one of the biggest barriers to successful change with today's busy world. Be aware that changes in this area might be the best place to start to allow the rest to happen.

Summary

- Energy can be physical, mental, emotional or spiritual.

- Your working life should draw from all four sources.

- Ensure your personal life is also physically energising, emotionally fulfilling, mentally stimulating and spiritually aligned!

- Work out what or who you need to support you.

- Have your vision somewhere in sight so that you can refer to it frequently when times get tough. Who would you be at your best?

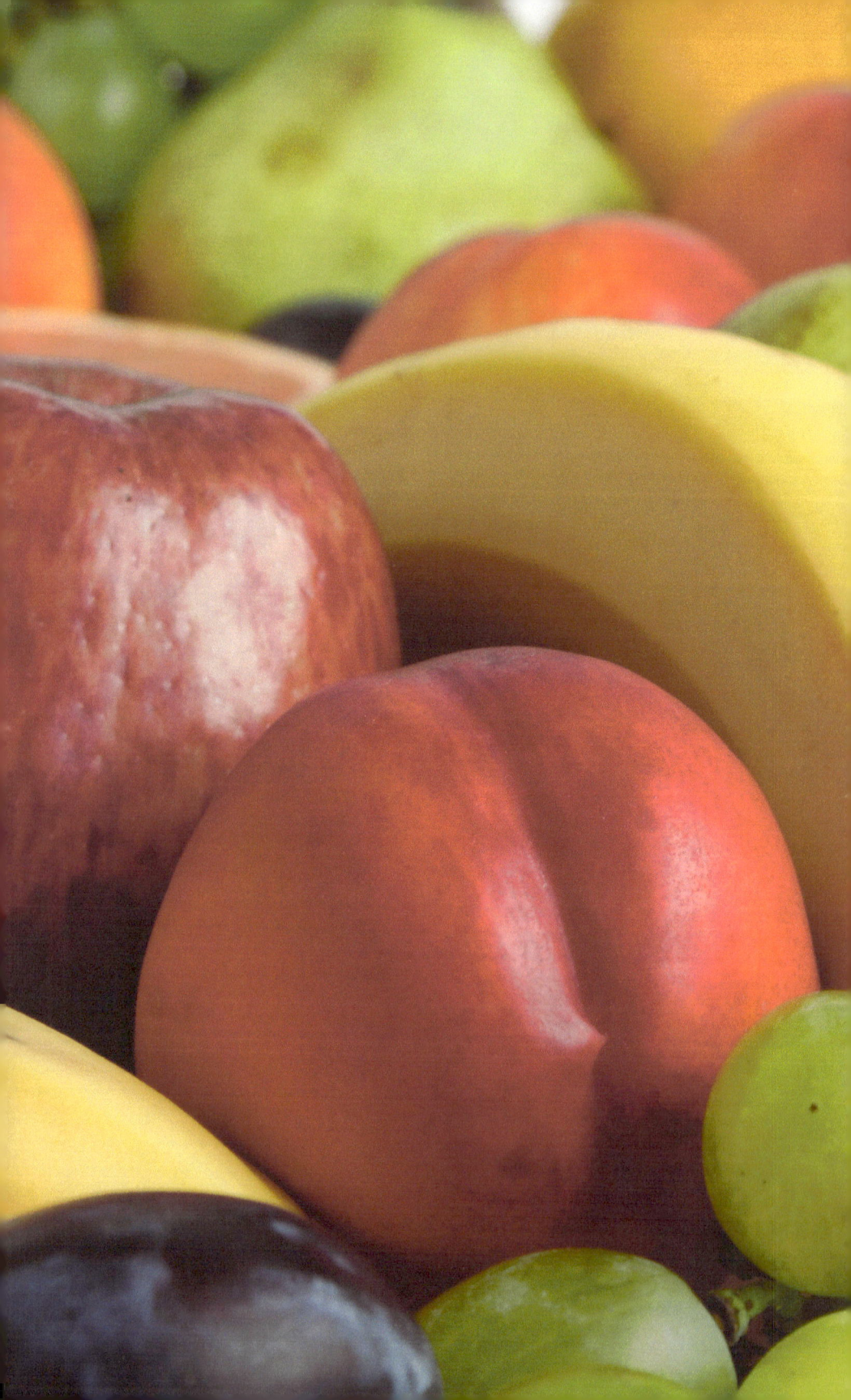

Final word

Being your own coach doesn't mean you do this in isolation. The process of asking for support may begin a lifestyle change itself – opening up different ways of relating – especially if you are someone who would normally prefer to do just about anything than ask someone for help.

That aside, there is an amazing opportunity here to develop a new relationship with yourself. When you have experienced how reliable you can be; how encouraging; how caring in your confrontation of yourself; hen you witness all the integrity it takes to coach yourself to wellness, you will know that you will never let yourself down again. You really can rely on you.

"The spirit of self help is the root of all genuine growth in the individual."

Samuel Smiles, 1859

Appendices contents page:

- 10 recommended tests to have before beginning

- Rediscovering the real you through nutrition and lifestyle

- 20 tips for beginning an exercise program

- N.E.A.T.

- Common lifestyle barriers to wellness

- Useful questionnaires

- Resource list – people and organisations who can help

- References

- Further reading

- Sample wellness plan

10 recommended tests to have before beginning

Dr John Lang, CEO JAKL

Dr. John Lang has worked in the area of executive health testing for many years and is now the CEO of JAKL focusing on culture, engagement, satisfaction, mental and physical health in the workforce.

Research consistently shows that those who "use" the health system will have better health outcomes than those who don't. This doesn't mean we need to become hypochondriacs, but to use the system judiciously. The following items should be the minimum requirements for your annual or biannual health check with your GP.

- Blood Pressure – It's quick, easy, accurate and cheap – and it could save your life. Much of the reduction in cardiovascular disease risk in the past half century is due to better management of hypertension. BP is a silent risk factor; unlike being overweight, unfit, stressed or a smoker, you can't self assess BP. You need your doctor for this one.

- Blood Cholesterol – This is the other silent risk factor. And don't stop at cholesterol; get your HDLs, LDLs and triglycerides done as well. The same blood specimen can be used for all these tests, and knowing all of them is helpful for determining overall risk.

- Blood Glucose –Approximately 1.6 million Australians have type 2 diabetes; 800,000 of them are undiagnosed (because they haven't been tested). Don't be one of them.

- Waist-Hip Ratio – This test is three to five times better at predicting cardiovascular disease risk than BMI (which incorrectly assumes

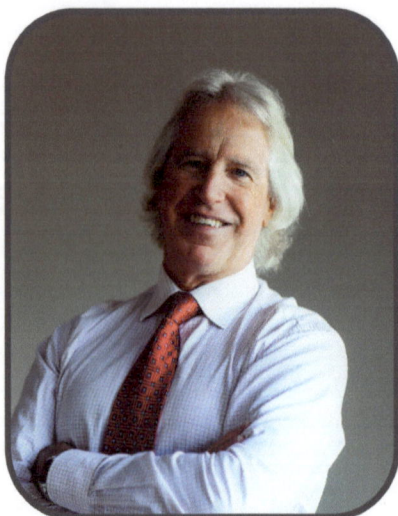

all excess weight to be fat).

- Skin Check – Almost 1000 Australians die each year from melanoma because they fail to check up on a darkening freckle or mole.

- K10 – A test for stress/anxiety/depression. The escalating prevalence of these conditions, which have a propensity to destroy quality of life, suggests the K10 test, or a similar psychometric test, should be considered as part of a regular check up.

- Mammogram – Women aged between 50 and 69 should have a mammogram every two years. About one in every 10 Australian women will develop breast cancer at some stage in their life. For almost one in four it will be fatal. If you have a family history, talk to your doctor about starting to screen earlier.

- Pap Smear – Any woman who has had sex (and who hasn't had a hysterectomy) should have a Pap test every two years. The new vaccine, Gardasil , will eventually result in a massive decline in the incidence of cervical cancer, but until then, screening is still prudent as two out of every three women diagnosed with this cancer will not survive it.

- PSA (Prostate Specific Antigen) – For men over 50, this test may be useful in the detection of prostate cancer (which affects one in 10 men). Doing the test on younger men results in an imbalance between the false positive and true positive results, which can cause anxiety and often lead to unnecessary follow up procedures.

- Bowel Cancer Check – One in 17 men and one in 26 women in Australia develop colorectal cancer. It is the second most prevalent cancer in both males and females – and has a 40 per cent mortality rate. Unlike the previous test for blood in the faeces which required a stool specimen to be taken to your GP for laboratory testing, these days a more sensitive test is available. You get the "kit" from your GP, take it home and just dip the small brush in the toilet water after a bowel motion, dab the wet brush onto a collection sheet and post it off to the lab in the mail. The test should be done every two years after age 50, unless advised otherwise by your doctor.

Rediscovering the real you through nutrition and lifestyle

Over many years of working with clients who are in different states of wellness, recovering from illness or suffering long term effects of poor health, there are five basic philosophies that have helped them move quickly towards better health.

1. **Eat whole food:** You can't go wrong - as much as possible eat whole goods. When you do that you may never need to understand those complicated food labels.

2. **Eat when you are hungry:** If you are hungry all the time it may be because you have too many refined carbs in your diet. Refined carbs are not nourishing and you and your body deserve the best nourishment.

3. **Chew your food** - You really need your digestive enzymes to support your digestion and gut microbiota. They are encouraged by chewing. Also great for your jaw, teeth and the muscle tone in your face.

4. **Lifestyle habits such as excerise, relaxation and sleep** are just as important when it comes to achieving your ideal weight. Stress hormones in the body activate inflammation in your body and can cause you to covert sugars/carbs into fat or resist fat loss.

5. **He who is most flexible WINS.** Be kind to yourself - sometimes life (or holiday season) gets in the way of best intentions. A little bit of pre planning goes a long way.

Developing a Program with your coach

The best way to rediscover a healthy weight and nutrition for you, is to be flexible in your approach within the boundaries of your goals. The greatest success comes from a plan that you can stick to long term.

A food journal is a great way to discover patterns in your eating that may not be serving you. You can change those patterns.

Are you a data driven person or do you like to be creative and free flowing? Do you like to keep a food journal? Create that type of plan with your coach that suits you

Build flexibility into the plan with your coach. There is always more than one way to achieve success.

"For a full copy of Linda's article, email info@wellnesscoachingaustralia.com.au with "Further book information" in the heading and we will send you the remaining information from the appendices."

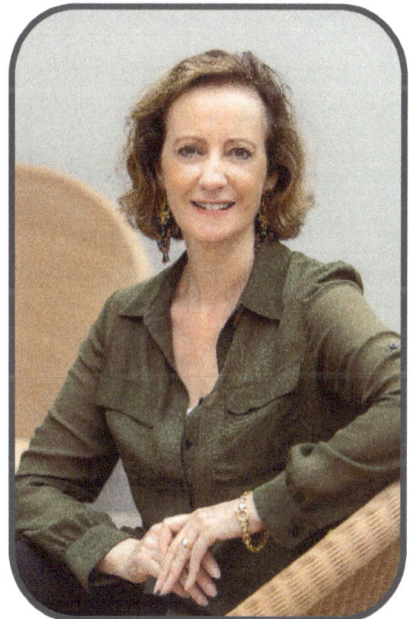

Linda Funnell-Milner
Functional Nutritionist
Clinical Hypnotherapist
Board Certified Health & Wellness Coach

20 tips for beginning an exercise program

Michael James, Personal Trainer
www.primal-fitness.com.au

- Sign up for a charity run/walk event
- Buy new training apparel
- Join a gym
- Arrange to walk RSPCA dogs
- Organise a training buddy or group
- Sign on with a personal trainer
- Coach a junior sport team
- Invest in a good pair of running shoes
- Re-work your schedule to include regular sessions for training
- Learn what foods you need to eat to have energy to exercise
- Get a health assessment
- Watch an inspirational movie/documentary
- Set small, achievable fitness goals
- Go roller-blading
- Go on a learn-to-surf safari
- Write down all the active pursuits you have enjoyed over the years
- Source your local bush walking club and join
- Talk to people who train and ask them why they do it
- Take the stairs
- Walk to work

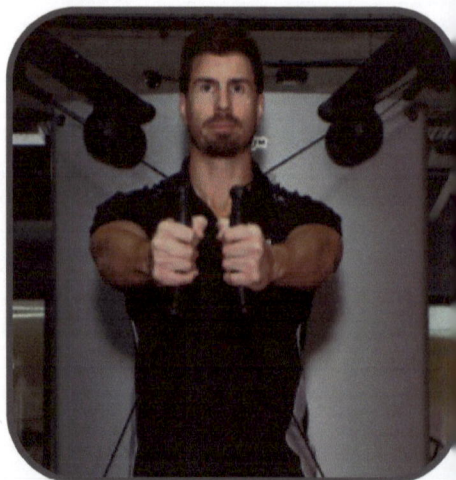

N.E.A.T. – What we need to know about movement

Dr. Paul Batman

Dr. Paul Batman has worked in health, fitness and sport for over 40 years. Known as the Inactivity Specialist, Paul has presented at international conventions and conducted lectures, workshops in many countries throughout the world. Paul has written over a hundred articles on all aspects health and fitness and authored or co-authored 10 books.

We know that inactivity is a killer. We are well educated about the risks of a sedentary lifestyle. So why is it that if more people are better educated about exercise and fitness than ever before, there are more fitness professionals working in the industry and there are more people attending fitness centres in greater numbers that the fitness industry in its present form is having limited success?

To reduce the current pandemic of physical inactivity there is now a need to promote physical activities that can be accessed, enjoyed and sustained by a greater number of people throughout their lifetime regardless of their socioeconomic backgrounds.

The emphasis should now be on interacting with our environment by "walking often, running sometimes and moving in different ways throughout our waking day in all aspects of our life… not just for 30-60 minutes per day". We need to "create a lifestyle inclusive of physical activity" in addition to participation in a structured more formal exercise program.

Dr Paul has valuable information to share on how we need to understand the concept of Non-Exercise Activity Thermogenesis (NEAT). For people who do not wish to engage in high intensity intermittent exercise sessions, making changes to their lifestyles can be hugely beneficial to their health.

NON-EXERCISE ACTIVITY THERMOGENESIS (NEAT)

NEAT is defined as a group of non-exercise behaviours that contribute to energy expenditure but fall below usual measurement of moderate-to-vigorous physical activity. Physical activity can be subdivided into energy expended in exercise and energy expended in non-exercise activity (NEAT).

This form of thermogenesis can account for a substantial proportion of daily energy expenditure, usually more than the sum of daily moderate-to-vigorous activities.

THE METABOLIC HEALTH CONSEQUENCES OF NEAT

Increasing the daily NEAT activity can result in a dramatic improvement in a person's overall health by reducing obesity risk factors, including percent body fat, body mass index, cholesterol, the HDL/LDL ratio and blood plasma triglycerides.

STRATEGIES TO PROMOTE AND IMPLEMENT NEAT

Occupation and leisure time are the two principal time frames that need to be targeted for promoting individual NEAT. Several strategies can be used to guide NEAT-based interventions that are aimed at increasing the amount of time spent standing or in ambulation.

These include:

- **Select standing and ambulating behaviours that are easy and enjoyable.**
- **Use self-monitoring to increase awareness.**

  This may be monitoring of sedentary activities like time spent watching TV or alternatively it may be monitoring of behavioural changes that are made.

- **Modify specific seated behaviours so they can be performed standing.**

  For example, if a person wants to play hand held computer games, then they could choose to do so standing.

- **Use sedentary behaviours to reinforce physically active behaviours.**

  For example, if a person wishes to watch TV then the can only do so if they have met their daily activity goals.

- **Identify behavioural substitutes.**

  This involves the person selecting an activity they enjoy and can perform instead of a sedentary one.

We are including a link to more detailed information on this relatively new and vital area to help both health and wellness coaches and community understand that there may be a different approach to the way we view "exercise".

This is a mere taster of this important aspect of healthy lifestyle. For more information, email us at info@wellnesscoachingaustralia.com.au or visit Dr. Paul's website http://www.drpaulbatman.com.au

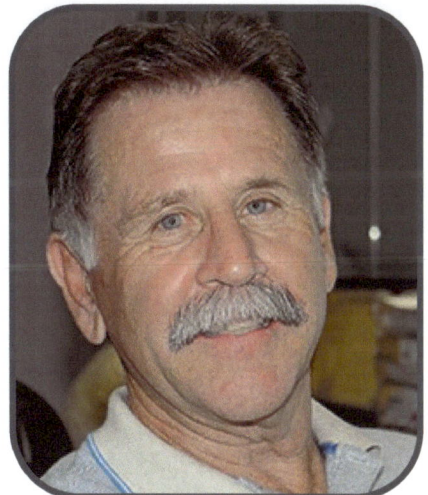

Common Lifestyle barriers to wellness

We live in complex times. Our state of wellness is affected by many things. Over the years, exercise and nutrition have been the main focus for change and recommended by the health professionals whose business it is to keep us healthy.

Yet they are now only two factors that affect people's sense of being well. Many things come into play and can be common barriers that often interlink with each other to contribute to disease and "dis-ease" of life.

They include:

- Sleep patterns
- Drug and alcohol use
- Personal organisation
- Financial wellness
- Stress and anxiety

Sometimes we need to create new habits in these areas to enable new behaviour to arise in others. We sometimes refer to them as "Foundation Habits". Get one thing working well and others will follow. E.g. stop smoking and the desire to exercise often increase.

It is very important for each of us to consider what could possibly be behind our undesirable routine.

- Are we suffering from stress and anxiety because of unrealistic expectations we place on ourselves?
- Is our sleep affected because of the tendency to consume too much alcohol, thinking that this will wipe away the stress of the day?
- Are we overwhelmed by the amount of responsibilities we have and our inability to organise our lives in a way that we allows us to manage (or reduce) these?

- Are our support circles diminishing because we lack time to keep meaningful connections with these people?
- Are we spending too much time locked to a screen and missing vital, healing time in nature?

These are just a few questions that can arise when we start to work with a coach or coach ourselves. Go to www.wellnesscoachingaustralia.com.au/Wellbeing-Studies/understanding-stress and you will find useful information on each of these in this module of study should you decide to undertake it.

Useful Questionnaires

(unless indicated otherwise, please email info@wellnesscoachingaustralia.com.au and request that a copy of this extra material be sent to you)

Adult Pre-Exercise Screen Tool

This is a questionnaire that can be used to determine safety of beginning an exercise program or advisability of getting a full medical check first.

Measuring Wellbeing

This questionnaire is a self inventory of various areas of wellness and is a great self awareness tool. It can also reveal your own readiness to create change in various areas of your life.

How Stressed are you?

This test will give you some idea about how much stress you deal with in your life right now. Go to the link below for an online assessment. https://psychcentral.com/quizzes/stress-test/

Common Sleep Disorders

A fact sheet on common sleep disorders and potential treatment approaches. Source: https://www.sleephealthfoundation.org.au

Resources

Organisations

- Fitness Australia – find a club or personal trainer in your area 1300 211 311
- National Heart Foundation – 1300 362 787 www.heartfoundation.org.au
- Quitline – 13 7848
- Diabetes Australia – worried you may be at risk? National Office (02) 6232 3800
- Beyond Blue – If you need support with severe anxiety or depression 1300 224 636

Coaching Support

Wellness coach or Wellness Coach training
– contact Wellness Coaching Australia
+61 2 8006 9055 info@wellnesscoachingaustralia.com.au
www.wellnesscoachingaustralia.com.au (see final page)

Bush walking

National Parks Association of NSW (02) 9299 0000

Cycling

Cycling Australia: 02 9644 3002

Coach Training

Wellness Coaching Australia

- Level 1,2 3 in Health and Wellness Coaching
- Professional Certificate in Health and Wellness Coaching
- Diploma in Health and Wellness Coaching - (10641NAT) - will be offered by a registered RTO and delivered and assessed by WCA.

Courses approved for graduates to sit for National Board Certification (Medical Board of Examiners in the U.S.)

For more information contact
info@wellnesscoachingaustralia.com.au
Tel: 02 8006 9055

References

Australia's Health 2006 - The tenth biennial health report of the Australian Institute of Health and Welfare AIHW Cat No. Aus 73

http:www.authentichappiness.sas.upenn.edu

Collins, D. & Lapsley, H. (2002). Counting the cost: estimates of the social costs of drug abuse in Australia in 1998–99. National Drug Strategy Monograph Series no. 49.Canberra: Department of Health and Ageing

Cycle of Change model adapted from Prochaska and Diclemente (1982).

Further reading

Arloski, M. (2007) *Wellness Coaching for Lasting Lifestyle Change*, Minnesota: Whole Person Associates, Inc.

Brown, B. (2017) *Braving the Wilderness*. London: Vermilion

Fredrickson, B. (2009) *Positivity*. New York: Three Rivers Press

Grant, A. and Green, J. (2001) *It's Your Life. What Are You Going To Do With It?* London: Pearson Education.

Grant, A. M., & Greene, J. (2003). *Coaching Yourself: When It's You That Needs to Change*. In R. Stock (Ed.), Get Ahead; Give a Damm (pp. 45-51). London: Pearson Education.

Grant A.M. and Greene J. (2005) *Coach Yourself at Work*, Sydney: ABC Books.

Greene, J. and Grant, A. M. (2003) *Solution-focused Coaching: Managing People in a Complex World*. London: Momentum Press

Grant, A. M. and Greene, J. (2001) *Coach Yourself: Make Real Change in Your Life*. London: Momentum Press.

Lang, J. (2002) *Re: Life*, Pearson Education Limited,.

Loehr, J and Schwartz, T (2003) *The Power of Full Engagement*, Sydney: Allen & Unwin.

McKay, H.(2013) *The Good Life*. Australia: Pan Macmillan

Prochaska, J., Norcross, J. and Diclemente, C. (1994; 2002) *Changing for Good*. New York, NY: Harper Collins/Quill.

Seligman, M. (2002) *Authentic Happiness: Using the New Positive Psychology to Realize Your Potential for Lasting Fulfillment*, New York: Free Press.

Seligman, M. (2012) *Flourish*. Australia: Random House

McKay, M. and Fanning, P. (1992) *Self Esteem*. (2nd Ed.), Oakland, Ca: New Harbinger Publications.

SAMPLE WELLNESS PLAN

Wellness Vision

My vision is to lose weight and get to somewhere between 60 and 62 kg. I want to increase my fitness and make exercise a regular discipline for myself.

There are many reasons why I want to achieve these things:

- To be seen as a healthy person
- To be a good role model for my kids
- To maximise my quality of life as I get older
- If I can achieve these things, I may then have the confidence to take on some new area of study and grow in my professional life

Some of the obstacles are:

- Cooking for the kids and eating food that I know I shouldn't be eating
- Four daughters' commitments and need to transport them
- Boredom with existing exercise program
- Guilt over not putting the kids first

My ideas for some strategies include:

- Go to bed earlier so not so tired and can exercise in the morning
- Get my partner involved in some exercise-based activity with me
- Choose from variety of classes at the gym
- Swim with a friend

My strengths or what I have going for me include:

- A supportive partner who also wants to lose weight

- Time – working hours and kids going to their Dad
- I enjoy exercise
- The place I live – great place to exercise
- My gym membership
- The choices I have – running, walking, cycling, gym, dancing etc.
- My energy and enthusiasm for life
- My values around health

My three-month goals:

Month started: February

- I will be doing a cardio workout on 3–4 days per week
  Comment: at a "huff and puff" level for at least 30 minutes

Nutrition:

- I will be eating a healthier diet that will consist of 3-4 servings of fruit and vegetables a day and dessert only twice a week.
- I will be drinking 5 glasses of water per day
- I will be having alcohol on no more than two week nights and at weekends, being Friday and Sunday. I will drink no more than 2 drinks when I have alcohol.

My next week's goals: (starting 14th Feb)

Exercise:

I will do the following exercise program:

Mon: Jog – 30 minutes on my own

Comment: speed not important, intensity higher than walk/jog

Tues: Pump/Body Jam

Thurs: Dancing

Sat: RPM/Swimming

Comment: Substitute alternative exercise or day if have to

Nutrition:

I will keep a log of food, I will have a light lunch (and exercise)
Comment: note size of meals and how often I eat them rather than every item of food.

I will record alcohol in log.

On late shift I will have light lunch and take small healthy snack
Comment: can have dinner with partner at end of day.

Wellness Coaching Australia

Wellness Coaching Australia is Australia's leading coach training organisation in the emerging field of Health and Wellness Coaching. Founded in 2006 by Fiona Cosgrove, Wellness Coaching Australia has trained thousands of students through its gold standard certification programs, short courses and workshops. As Australia's first Health and Wellness Coach training organisation to be an approved training provider by the National Board for Health and Wellness Coaching (US), students know they are undertaking the highest level of training standards - globally.

JOIN OUR TRIBE

Turn your passion for health, wellness and helping others into an enriching profession by choosing to train with Wellness Coaching Australia. There are many levels of learning options available, whether it be attending a workshop or completing a short course to upskill, or completing a full certification course with the view to working professionally as a Health and Wellness Coach.

Workshops, Seminars and Short Courses

Wellness Coaching Australia offers a range of workshops, seminars and short courses in the areas of coaching, health, physical activity, nutrition and wellness. These are ideal for those starting their Health and Wellness Coaching journey and looking for personal and professional development courses as well as practitioners already working in the health and wellness field and are looking to upskill and add coaching communication skills to their existing work.

Certification Programs

If you are passionate about supporting individuals in healthy lifestyles and empowering them to achieve their health and wellness goals, then training to become a professional Health and Wellness Coach is an enriching journey both professionally and personally . Wellness Coaching Australia offers a number of certificate programs – training of the highest quality. These programs include:

- Professional Certificate in Health and Wellness Coaching
- Nationally Accredited - Diploma of Health and Coaching (10641NAT) - will be offered by a registered RTO and delivered and assessed by WCA.

For more information on Wellness Coaching Australia's training programs, visit www.wellnesscoachingaustralia.com.au or email info@wellnesscoachingaustralia.com.au

Take the next step – get the workbook

Start on your journey to change with the *Coach Yourself to Wellness Workbook*. Also by Fiona Cosgrove, this easy-to-use book of exercises and action steps is designed to help you document your coaching journey. Whether you are coaching yourself or you are using a coach/trainer, the Coach Yourself to Wellness Workbook will provide structure and a concrete format to follow. Don't fall short of your goals purely because you lack a well-prepared foundation for success.

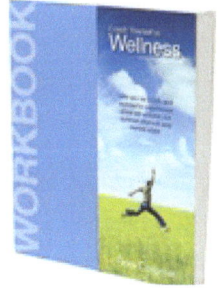

To order your copy, visit www.wellnesscoachingaustralia.com.au

www.ingramcontent.com/pod-product-compliance
Lightning Source LLC
Chambersburg PA
CBHW040931030426
42334CB00007B/113